COLON &
RECTAL
CANCER

A Patient's Guide to Treatment

PAUL RUGGIERI, M.D.

Addicus Books
Omaha, Nebraska

An Addicus Nonfiction Book

ISBN 1-886039-51-8
Cover design by Peri Poloni
Illustrations by Jack Kusler
Typography by Linda Dageforde

This book is not intended to serve as a substitute for a physician, nor does the author intend to give medical advice contrary to that of an attending physician.

Library of Congress Cataloging-in-Publication Data
Ruggieri, Paul, 1959-
    Colon and rectal cancer : a patient's guide to treatment / Paul
Ruggieri.
        p. cm.
Includes bibliographical references and index.
    ISBN 1-886039-51-8
    1. Colon (Anatomy)—Cancer. 2. Rectum—Cancer. I. Title.
RC280.C6 R84 2001
616.99'4347—dc21

                                                              2001000177

Addicus Books, Inc.
P.O. Box 45327
Omaha, Nebraska 68145
Web site: http://www.AddicusBooks.com
Printed in the United States of America
10 9 8 7 6 5 4 3 2 1

To all those who have survived cancer. Thank you for teaching us about courage, will, and determination in defeating one of life's most formidable foes.

Acknowledgments

I would first like to thank all my patients—past and present—for the privilege of being involved in their care. I'd also like to acknowledge my patients' family members. Their love, understanding, and support is so vital for ensuring a healthy recovery.

I would also like to thank Christine Gillespie, R.N., both for her care of my colorectal cancer patients and for her input on this book. I wish to thank Diane Peckham, R.N., Certified Wound, Ostomy, and Continence Nurse, for her expertise on the care of a colostomy. I also acknowledge Amit Choksi, M.D., Gastroenterologist, for his professionalism and efforts in helping people diagnosed with colorectal cancer. His friendship will always be very special to me.

This book would not have been possible without the efforts of all those involved at Addicus Books. I especially thank Rod Colvin for his uncompromising focus and drive for perfection. I appreciate the editorial efforts of Bobbie Hasselbring and the illustrative works of Jack Kusler and Peri Poloni.

Finally, I would like to thank Larry Connors for his inspiration and my parents for their courage and support.

Contents

Introduction

Has your life suddenly been interrupted by an unexpected diagnosis of cancer? Has someone close to you just been diagnosed with the disease? Your first reaction may be shock, denial, or anger. It doesn't seem fair that you're suddenly forced to come face-to-face with a life-threatening disease. You may be thinking, "Why me? Why my family?" Your reactions and feelings are normal and understandable.

It may be of comfort to know that you are not alone. Cancer isn't something that just affects other people. Unfortunately, today cancer affects *everyone* directly or indirectly. This is especially true of colorectal cancer.

Colorectal cancer—cancer of the colon and rectum—is much more common than most other cancers. It is the second leading cause of cancer death in the United States. Among people who don't smoke, colorectal cancer is the number one cause of cancer death. Colorectal cancer doesn't discriminate. It affects famous people and ordinary individuals alike.

In the past, colorectal cancer was difficult to understand and even more difficult to talk about. However, that has changed, thanks to the educational efforts of high-profile people like network television personality Katie Couric, whose husband died of colorectal cancer. People today are talking about colorectal cancer and getting screening tests that can diagnose it early. The best news is, you can actually *prevent* colorectal cancer by making healthy lifestyle choices, knowing your risk factors, and getting the proper screening tests. Even if you are diagnosed with colorectal cancer, treatments today are more effective than ever.

My purpose in writing this book is twofold. The first is to help you understand how to keep this disease from ever affecting you and your loved ones. Prevention is the best weapon we have in our arsenal to fight colorectal cancer. This book will help you understand what annual screening involves, how it saves lives, and how it can prevent the disease. My second goal is to calm your fears, reassure you, and answer all the questions that invariably come with a diagnosis of colorectal cancer.

When you or someone you love is being treated for cancer, the doctors, the tests, and the operations often feel overwhelming and frightening. The information in this book will help you understand your disease and help replace your fear with knowledge. It will guide you through the process of diagnosis and testing, questions to ask your doctor, the treatment options, and what you can look forward to for the rest of your life.

Thanks to the educational efforts of many people whose lives have been touched by colorectal cancer, people are realizing that

Introduction

this common disease is preventable, treatable, and curable. My hope is this book will add to those efforts and help make your personal experience a better one.

The bravest are surely those who have the clearest
Vision of what is before them, glory and danger alike,
And yet notwithstanding, go but to meet it.
—Thucydides 404 b.c.

1

The Colon and Colorectal Cancer

Colorectal cancer is a potentially deadly, abnormal growth of cells in the colon and/or rectum, a long, muscular tube that is part of your digestive system. Unfortunately, colorectal cancer is all too common. It affects more than 130,000 people each year in the United States. It is the second leading cause of death due to cancer in this country, second only to lung cancer. One out of eight deaths due to cancer are caused by colorectal cancer. Still, the disease is very curable if detected early. In fact, in 75 percent of new cases, the cancer has not yet spread to other organs.

Colorectal cancer affects both men and women. Women develop more colon cancer than men, but fewer rectal cancers. In the United States, the American Cancer Society estimates that each year more than 50,000 women and 43,000 men are diagnosed with colon cancer; more than 16,000 women and 20,000 men are diagnosed with rectal cancer.

Colorectal cancer is a disease of Western civilization. It is not common in Far Eastern countries, such as Japan or China. This fact may have to do with our diet and the environment, something we'll talk more about in this chapter.

Anatomy of the Colon and Rectum

To better understand colorectal cancer and how it impacts your body, it's important to know what the colon and rectum are and how they function. The colon and rectum are important parts of your *gastrointestinal (GI) tract.* The gastrointestinal tract includes your *mouth, esophagus, stomach, duodenum* (first part of your small intestine), *small intestine, colon* (large intestine), *rectum,* and *anus.* This system digests food, absorbs nutrients, and excretes waste.

The colon (also called the large bowel) is a hollow, tube-like organ five to six feet long and up to five inches in diameter. Entirely separate from the small intestine, it begins where the small intestine ends.

The colon sits inside the *abdominal cavity* and is divided into segments that have different names based on their location and the direction in which each moves waste (fecal) material. The *ileocecal valve* separates the small intestine from the colon. This valve opens and closes, controlling the flow of waste fluid into the colon. The first part of the colon is a pouch called the *cecum.* The next segment is the *ascending* or *right colon,* located on the right side of the abdomen and situated up toward the liver. The *transverse colon* crosses over the midsection of the abdomen. Down from the *spleen* on the left side of the abdominal cavity is the *descending* or *left colon.* The left colon leads into the *sigmoid colon,* an S-shaped section that connects to the rectum. The rectum is the last six to ten inches of colon as it exits out the anus.

The colon consists of four different layers of tissue. The innermost layer, the *mucosa,* is in direct contact with fecal material as it moves through the colon and is responsible for much of the colon's function. The thin mucosa is composed of specialized cells that are in a constant state of flux, continually dying, sloughing off, and being replaced with new cells. The layer beneath the mucosa is the *submucosa.* It's a specialized layer of cells that helps support the mucosa. The next layer of tissue is the *muscularis propria.* The muscle cells in this layer give strength to the colon wall and cause the contractions that push fecal material along the colon. The outermost layer is the *serosa.* The serosal cells add more support to the colonic wall and act as a barrier, protecting the colon from any outside invading disease.

How the Colon and Rectum Work

The primary job of the colon is to manage and remove solid waste. It also absorbs water and *electrolytes,* such as sodium and potassium, which enables cells to function and replenish.

When you eat, food spends several hours in the stomach getting broken down (digested) into tiny pieces. It is then propelled into the first portion of the small intestine (duodenum). Once the nutrients are absorbed in the small intestine, the remaining liquid (*chyme)* enters the colon through the ileocecal valve. By the time the liquid enters the first part of the colon (cecum), it contains no nutrients and is pure waste product. In the colon, this waste liquid is slowly propelled toward the rectum. Over a four- to six-hour period, the liquid moves through the colon and the mucosal cells absorb water from it. The colon can absorb nearly two gallons of water a day. The end product is the solid waste (feces) we excrete.

The rectum, the last six to ten inches of colon that is continuous with the anus, is located deep behind the *pubic bone* and *urinary bladder*. Its primary job is to store processed fecal material before it is removed from the body. Once there is enough fecal material in the rectum, sensory nerves tell the brain it is time to have a bowel movement. Unlike the rest of the colon, the walls of the rectum are primarily composed of muscle cells that propel the fecal material out of the body.

How Colorectal Cancer Starts

Normally, cells throughout our bodies divide and reproduce, repairing and replacing worn-out tissue. However, sometimes this growth process goes out of control and the cells begin to multiply rapidly. Cancer is an overgrowth of these abnormal cells.

Colorectal cancer starts in the inner lining of either the colon or rectum. The abnormal cells may grow uncontrollably without any early warning signs. Usually, they grow unnoticed until the mass they create reaches a size that causes symptoms or is detected by diagnostic tests. The entire process, from a single cell to a detectable cancerous tumor, can take up to twenty years. Most people have no idea a tumor is growing inside their colon or rectum unless they go for routine tests or start to experience symptoms.

Cancerous or Benign?

When talking about your condition, your doctor may use a number of terms. He or she may use the words *tumor, growth, mass, lesion,* and *neoplasm* interchangeably to refer to abnormal

Abdominal Organs

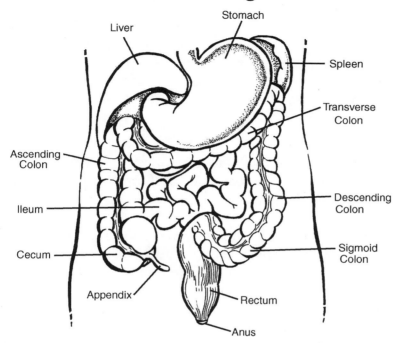

Liver
Stomach
Spleen
Transverse Colon
Ascending Colon
Descending Colon
Ileum
Cecum
Sigmoid Colon
Appendix
Rectum
Anus

tissue growth. A *polyp* is a special type of growth we'll talk about in greater detail in this chapter.

A tumor, growth, mass, lesion, neoplasm, or polyp in the colon or rectum can either be benign or malignant. The word *benign* means noncancerous. The term *malignant* means cancerous—the kind of tissue that can invade and destroy normal tissue. When a tumor is discovered in the colon or rectum, it is not called malignant until cells from a biopsy prove it. The decision whether a tumor is malignant or benign is made only after the biopsied tumor cells are examined under the microscope.

A growth can also be labeled *precancerous*. This means the growth contains suspicious-looking cells when viewed under the microscope, so it cannot be called benign. Yet these cells do not meet the criteria to be called malignant. If precancerous cells are not removed or treated, they can develop into a true cancer that can spread. Once a cancer has spread to other parts of the body, it is said to have *metastasized*.

Polyps

Polyps are small growths that can occur anywhere along the gastrointestinal tract. They can also be found in other organs of the body, such as the gallbladder, the nose, or even on the vocal cords.

Polyps are very common in the colon and rectum. They occur more frequently in people over age fifty. Studies estimate that 50 percent of the U.S. population has polyps in the colon and/or rectum.

Polyps form over a long period of time—five to ten years. They are caused by genetic changes in the cells lining the inside of the colon. Often people are unaware that polyps exist in their colon until the polyps grow large enough to cause symptoms, such as pain or bleeding.

Colorectal polyps may be malignant or benign. Most polyps removed by doctors are benign; cancer cells are present in only about 1 percent of polyps. However, benign polyps can grow and turn into cancer. The larger the polyp, the greater chance it will be cancerous.

Changing a benign, noncancerous polyp into a malignant one involves genetic changes, called mutations, which evolve over a prolonged period of time. These mutations must occur in certain genes at certain times and in a specific sequence. This is why only 1 percent of polyps are cancerous despite a potential 50 percent of the older population having them. As mutations occur, a noncancerous polyp may be transformed into a precancerous polyp, and finally into a cancerous polyp. Cancerous polyps are dangerous and can spread to other organs. This is why the screening tests on the colon, discussed in chapter 11, are important. If a colorectal polyp is detected and removed before it becomes cancerous, colorectal cancer can be prevented.

Types of Polyps

Several types of benign, precancerous, and cancerous polyps may occur in the colon. The types are defined by their size and by how the cells appear under the microscope.

Benign Polyps

Hyperplastic

This common type of benign polyp is small, the size of a pea. It consists of a dense cluster of normal cells with no microscopic abnormalities. It is a totally benign polyp with no potential to become cancerous.

Inflammatory

This type of benign polyp is also small and made up of a dense population of inflamed cells commonly associated with inflammatory diseases of the colon, including ulcerative colitis and Crohn's disease.

Hamartoma

This type of benign polyp is also small and found in patients with genetically inherited polyp syndromes. These polyps are frequently numerous and scattered throughout the colon.

Precancerous Polyps

Precancerous polyps, or *adenomas*, can be divided into three categories.

Tubular

This type of polyp can grow to several inches in diameter and is made up of tube-shaped cells. Tubular polyps are generally considered premalignant, with the potential to turn cancerous if not removed. There is a 5 percent chance of a tubular polyp becoming cancerous.

Tubulovillous

This type of polyp can grow to four to five inches in diameter. They are made up of a combination of tubular cells and villous cells, which appear as a cluster of fingerlike projections. These polyps have a higher potential—20 percent—to turn into cancer because of the presence of villous cells.

Villous

This type of premalignant polyp can also grow to four to five inches in diameter but is made up solely of villous cells. Villous polyps have the greatest potential to become malignant, up to a 40 percent chance.

Cancerous Polyps

When a polyp is determined to be cancerous, the cancer may be classified as a *carcinoma in situ* or as an *adenocarcinoma*.

Carcinoma in situ

Here, a polyp contains cancer cells at the beginning of their life cycle. The malignant cells are contained to the polyp and have no potential to spread to other organs.

Adenocarcinoma

The most common cancer of the colon, adenocarcinomas have the potential to spread outside the polyp to other organs.

Characteristics of Cancerous Polyps

Several factors influence whether a colorectal polyp is malignant. These factors include the size of the polyp, its shape, location in the colon, and the presence or absence of microscopic changes to the DNA—the cell's "blueprint" for growth.

Polyps run in my family. I was not aware that they could turn into cancer if not removed.

Carol, 52
Patient

Size

The larger the polyp, the greater the chance of it being cancerous. For instance, a polyp less than ½ inch (or 1 cm) has a less than 10 percent chance of being cancerous. However, polyps more than 1 inch in diameter (2 cm) can have a 20 to 30 percent chance of being cancerous. It is important to remove polyps early so they cannot grow to sizes that increase the potential for cancer.

Shape

The general shape of a colorectal polyp also influences the potential of it being cancerous. Polyps that are located on a stalk, with the stalk attached to the inner lining of the colon wall, are easy to remove and less likely to be cancerous. However, polyps that are very broad-based are more difficult to remove and more likely to be cancerous. Broad-based polyps are called sessile polyps.

Location

The location of a polyp is also important. Cancerous polyps are more commonly found in the sigmoid colon and rectum than in the right, transverse, or left colon. It has been estimated that more than 50 percent of cancerous polyps are located in the sigmoid colon and rectum.

Dysplasia

Dysplasia is the medical term used to describe the genetic changes (mutations) observed in the DNA of polyp cells. When cells are dysplastic their centers (nuclei) are misshapen. The more dysplastic changes, the greater the chance of finding cancer cells. Dysplastic changes lead to carcinoma in situ, and this leads to invasive cancer if not detected.

Many factors influence whether a colorectal polyp has the potential to turn cancerous. These factors are all considered when a doctor finds a polyp, biopsies or removes it, and decides whether further definitive treatment is necessary. The important point here is finding polyps early. Once found, your doctor can remove them before they ever become cancerous.

Are You at Risk for Colorectal Cancer?

What is your risk for developing colorectal cancer? Does your lifestyle and/or family genetics put you at increased risk? The answers to these questions are important in deciding how often you need to see your doctor for routine screening. There are several *risk factors* associated with colorectal cancer. Fortunately, many of them can be changed to decrease your risk.

No one knows exactly what causes colorectal cancer. However, doctors think genetic changes, coupled with dietary and environmental factors, play a major role in changing normal cells into cancerous cells.

Risk Factors for Colorectal Cancer

Having one or more of these risk factors increases the chance that you'll develop colorectal cancer sometime in your life.

- Family history/genetics
- Increasing age
- Personal history of precancerous polyps or colorectal cancer
- High-fat, high-meat diet
- Inflammatory bowel disease
- Smoking
- Obesity
- Physical inactivity
- Certain occupations

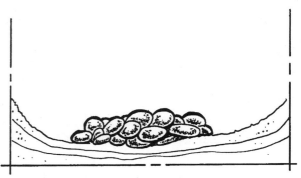

Broad-based, or sessile, polyps are more likely to be cancerous.

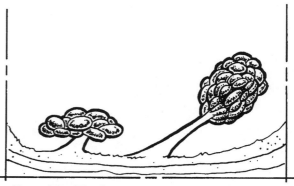

Examples of the "polyp on a stalk" are shown above. These polyps are less likely to be cancerous.

Family History/Genetics

A family history of colorectal cancer is the most important risk factor. Having someone in your family with colorectal cancer, particularly a first-degree relative (parent or sibling), puts you at a much higher risk than someone without a family history of the disease. If a second- degree relative (aunt, uncle, or cousin) has colorectal cancer, the risk is lower, but still higher than for no family history of the disease.

There is also increasing evidence that a family history of uterine, breast, and ovarian cancer may increase the risk for colorectal cancer. Knowing your family history is vital to understanding your risk and developing a screening plan with your doctor.

Several genetically inherited syndromes may predispose you to developing early colorectal cancer. If you or a member of your family is diagnosed with one of these syndromes, you're at higher risk. Fortunately, most of these syndromes are rare. However, they can be deadly if not diagnosed and treated early.

- Familial adenomatous polyposis (FAP) is an inherited disease that causes the formation of thousands of polyps along the entire gastrointestinal tract. These polyps form at an early age, and if left untreated, will turn cancerous before age 40. This syndrome is associated with cancers involving other organ systems, such as cancers of the liver, thyroid gland, and brain.

- Hereditary Nonpolyposis Colon Cancer (HNPCC) results in the formation of potentially cancerous polyps well before age 20.

- Turcot's syndrome links the formation of cancerous colorectal polyps with an aggressive form of brain cancer.

- Gardner's syndrome, similar to Turcot's, causes cancerous colorectal polyps and other organ cancers.
- Peutz-Jeghers syndrome and Cowden's syndrome are two genetic disorders that cause a polyp to form in the colon. Both diseases may also increase the risk for developing colorectal cancer later in life.

Age

Anyone at any age can develop colorectal cancer. However, more than 90 percent of the people diagnosed with colorectal cancer are over the age of 50. The average age of people diagnosed with colorectal cancer is close to 70.

If you're under age 40 and have no other risk factors, you're at very low risk for getting colorectal cancer. After age 50, however, population studies show that your risk increases dramatically. That's why routine checkups and screening for most people should start at age 50.

Personal History

If you have had colorectal polyps or have been treated for colorectal cancer in the past, you are at a much higher risk to redevelop either disease in the future. Follow-up tests after you have been treated for colorectal cancer can help minimize your risk.

Diet

What you eat affects your risk. A diet high in meat, high in saturated fats, and low in fiber (the so-called Western diet) places you at greater risk for developing colorectal cancer.

This is evident in studies of Japanese immigrants who come to the United States. The incidence of colorectal cancer in Japan is much lower. This is presumably due to the high-fiber, low-fat diet prevalent in Japan. However, when Japanese come to the United States and adopt a more Western diet, within two generations their risk of developing colorectal cancer is the same as ours.

The risk stems from potential cancer- causing agents, or carcinogens, that can form when the body ingests fatty acids and cholesterol. When fatty foods are cooked and processed, saturated fatty acids and cholesterol are broken down into potential cancer-causing by-products. Over time, these carcinogens interact with the cells lining the inside of the colon, damaging their DNA. The damaged (mutated) DNA can then greatly increase the potential of these cells to turn cancerous.

What we eat clearly influences our risk for colorectal cancer as well as many other cancers.
Lisa
Nutritionist

It is well known that a diet high in fiber can potentially reduce the risk for some diseases affecting the colon, including cancer. Fiber is thought to trap or dilute the cancer-causing agents ingested in our diet. Fiber also decreases the time ingested carcinogens interact with the lining of the colon by flushing them out quicker.

Inflammatory Bowel Disease

Two diseases that affect the lining of the colon are associated with an increased risk of colorectal cancer over time.

Ulcerative colitis causes inflammation of the inner layer of colon cells and results in chronic pain, bleeding, and diarrhea. It can affect an isolated segment of the colon or the entire organ. The cause of ulcerative colitis is not known and there is no effective medical cure. Surgery often is the only potential curative option, but it can't prevent the disease from coming back later in life. During the first ten years people have ulcerative colitis, the risk of developing colorectal cancer is low. However, after the first ten years, the risk increases 20 percent every ten years. Screening should start ten years after the initial diagnosis.

Crohn's disease also increases the risk for colorectal cancer. Like ulcerative colitis, Crohn's disease involves inflammation of the inner layer of the colon. It usually also involves other layers of the colon wall. Crohn's disease leads to abdominal pain, bleeding, infection, blockages, and diarrhea. The disease has no known cause and treatment can be difficult. The longer a person lives with Crohn's disease, the greater the risk for developing colorectal cancer.

Smoking

Studies by the American Cancer Society show that prolonged smoking can significantly increase your risk of dying from colorectal cancer. According to the data, if you have smoked for more than twenty years, your risk of dying from colorectal cancer can be increased 40 percent. It is now becoming clear that the more you smoke, the more you increase your risk of cancer. It is also becoming evident that the younger you start smoking, the greater your risk. This is true for both men and women.

Obesity, Physical Inactivity, and Certain Occupations

Several medical studies indicate that being overweight and physically inactive increase the risk for colorectal cancer. If you're very overweight, especially if you carry your excess weight around your waist, you're at increased risk for colorectal cancer. Some researchers suggest that excess fat changes metabolism (how the body converts food to energy) in a way that increases the growth of cells in the colon.

People who don't get a minimum amount of exercise are also at increased risk for colorectal cancer. Studies suggest that exercise, such as jogging or walking, may lower the risk for colorectal cancer. Exercise also has well-known benefits for the heart and lungs and helps control weight.

Certain occupations may put you at increased risk for colorectal cancer. Occupations involving asbestos exposure, such as shipyard, construction, and certain types of factory work, carry an increased risk for colorectal cancer as well as an increased risk for lung cancer.

Questions to Ask Your Doctor

- What are my risk factors for developing colorectal cancer?
- When should I start to be concerned about these risk factors?
- What can I do to minimize my risk?
- How can you as a doctor help minimize my risk?
- How can I change my diet to minimize my risk for colorectal cancer?

2

Symptoms of Colorectal Cancer

The symptoms of colorectal cancer can at times be very subtle or very obvious. Mild complaints may include abdominal pain, passing blood with bowel movements, or "just not feeling right." Early on, you may feel fine, not aware of the presence of a colorectal cancer. Frequently, a routine physical exam or abnormal blood tests can lead the doctor to suspect the presence of a colorectal cancer even when you have no symptoms and feel fine.

With colorectal cancer, the body often gives hints that something is wrong. Unfortunately, many people ignore the signs or pretend nothing is wrong. Many people are "too busy" to pay attention to their body's signals. They do not realize that a minor complaint like abdominal pain may signal the beginning of a cancer. Pretending a subtle body change is really "nothing to worry about" delays diagnosis of a potentially curable cancer. This denial may stem from the fear that the doctor may actually find something seriously wrong. Other people are embarrassed to talk about changes in bowel habits, an early warning sign for a growing cancer. This embarrassment can delay the diagnosis of a colorectal cancer and can greatly impact your chance for survival. Do not ignore your body's warning signs, particularly if you are at risk for colorectal cancer. The best chance to cure colorectal cancer is to diagnose it early, before it has spread.

Symptoms of Colorectal Cancer

Especially in the beginning, you may have some, all, or none of these symptoms. If you have any of these symptoms, see your doctor immediately.

- Change in bowel habits
- Rectal bleeding
- Sensation of needing a bowel movement
- Excess mucus secretion
- Chronic abdominal pain, bloating, fullness
- Decreased appetite
- Fatigue
- Weight loss

Change in Bowel Habits

A common early warning symptom of colorectal cancer is a subtle change in your bowel habits. Changes in your bowel pattern may include:

- Persistent loose stools
- Constipation
- Vague discomfort with bowel movements
- Pencil-thin stool

Be aware of these sudden changes and discuss them with your doctor. Do not delay in seeking your doctor's opinion on whether any of these changes are worrisome.

Rectal Bleeding

Passing bright red or dark blood is another warning symptom of colorectal cancer. This is especially true of cancers located in the left or sigmoid colon and the rectum. You may notice blood mixed in with stool or on the toilet paper. The blood mixed with stool may be dark, almost black, in color (called melena). The passing of bright red blood is called hematochezia. Passing blood may occur without pain. You may not even notice it if the blood loss is subtle and occurs slowly. Regardless of how often it occurs, if you are in the right age group and are at risk, get the problem checked out. Do not attribute any bleeding to a hemorrhoid problem and forget about it.

I thought my occasional bleeding was from hemorrhoids. I had no pain but my wife kept telling me to get a checkup. I was lucky because my cancer was found early and now I am fine.

Jason, 56
Survivor

Sensation of Needing a Bowel Movement

The urge to have a bowel movement is a common symptom in people diagnosed with a cancer of the rectum. It is a feeling of still needing to move your bowels despite just having done so. Doctors call this incomplete evacuation tenesmus. The feeling is caused by a tumor growing inside the rectum that takes up space and creates pressure. If you have this feeling, have it checked out by your doctor.

Excess Mucus Secretion

Some colorectal cancers, particularly those of the rectum, secrete excess mucus. It is seen with bowel movements and could be a sign of a growing rectal cancer.

Chronic Abdominal Pain, Bloating, Fullness

Most patients diagnosed with colorectal cancer experience very little abdominal pain prior to diagnosis. Pain is not a common warning symptom for this type of cancer, especially during its early stages. If the disease has spread beyond the colon or rectal wall into other organs, abdominal pain is common. Patients with abdominal pain usually describe it as dull, nagging, intermittent pain that doesn't go away. It generally does not occur during bowel movements.

> *My dad had colorectal cancer when he was 55, so this put me at a higher risk for getting the disease.*
> *Joseph, 45*
> *Patient*

Unfortunately, most people ignore this type of pain until it starts to impact their everyday activities. If you have recurrent pain, do not attribute it to an upset stomach, too much stress, food choices, or hope it will "just go away." If pain persists, get it checked by a physician.

Abdominal bloating, fullness, and distension that comes and goes may also signal a growing colorectal cancer. Sometimes people say they can feel a mass in their abdomen, a mass that was never there before. If you experience any of these symptoms, see your doctor.

Decreased Appetite, Fatigue, Weight Loss

Some people with colorectal cancer complain of not having an appetite, of losing weight despite eating, or of just not having any energy. Lack of appetite and weight loss are common symptoms, particularly if the cancer has spread. In people who have lost a significant amount of weight without trying to, the cancer has often spread to other organs. Lack of energy or fatigue may be caused by the slow, progressive loss of blood caused by the cancer. If you have these symptoms, you'll need tests to determine whether you have colorectal cancer.

Questions to Ask Your Doctor

- If I have occasional minor bleeding, when should I be concerned or have it checked out?
- If a symptom appears, how long should I wait before seeing a doctor?
- If I have one of the mentioned symptoms, does it mean I have cancer?
- When should I be concerned about prolonged constipation or diarrhea?
- Is there any way to know if a colorectal cancer is growing inside me?

3

Getting a Diagnosis

If you have any of the symptoms of colorectal cancer, it's important to see your doctor sooner rather than later. It might mean the difference between curing an early cancer or discovering the cancer has already spread. Fortunately, about 75 percent of colorectal cancers are detected early—before the cancer has spread to other parts of the body. How is it that so many cases are caught early? It takes a long time—sometimes years—for a colon cancer to grow through the colon wall; this expanse of times increases the likelihood that an individual will have a colon cancer screening test or seek medical attention for symptoms. Still, doctors cannot predict which cancers will have spread. Some smaller tumors may, for reasons not fully known, release cancer cells into the blood and to other organs. Other times, tumors may grow to a large size and yet not spread.

The five-year survival rate for people who are diagnosed and treated early is 90 percent. Once the cancer has spread to nearby organs or lymph nodes, that figure drops to 65 percent. When the cancer spreads to distant organs such as the lungs, the five-year survival rate is 8 percent. Clearly, early detection and diagnosis are the key to survival.

Let your doctor know about all your symptoms so that he or she can determine if they need further investigating. In many instances, your symptoms do not mean cancer. They often indicate a much less serious problem. However, you won't know this unless you get them checked out. Only your doctor can make a diagnosis, usually with the help of additional tests and a referral to a specialist.

Most people see their primary or family doctor first. This is where you should begin your colorectal cancer screening/diagnosis.

History and Physical Examination

During the first part of your office visit, your doctor will take a personal history and ask you about your symptoms. He or she will ask about changes in your bowel habits, the passing of blood, and if you've been having abdominal pain, weight loss, and/or decreased appetite. The doctor will want to know if you have any family history of colorectal cancer, including who and at what age close relatives were diagnosed with it. You may not know all the details of your family's medical history. Talk with relatives before you go to the doctor to make sure you have all the facts. A complete and accurate personal and family medical history can provide your doctor with important clues that can help diagnose your condition.

The second part of your office visit will include a physical examination. Your doctor will examine your entire body, focusing on certain aspects affected by colorectal cancer. If your doctor suspects cancer, he or she will look for such things as weight loss, a sign that the cancer may have spread to other organs. He or she will also be looking for *scleral icterus,* the medical term for yellowed or *jaundiced* eyes. This may mean the cancer has spread to your liver since it controls the production of a substance called *bilirubin.* If a cancer has spread to the liver, it can cause an increase of this substance in the blood, skin, and in the whites of the eyes.

Your doctor will examine your abdomen, looking for any fullness, masses, areas that are painful, or an enlarged liver. Any one of these can hint at the presence of a colorectal cancer or indicate another health problem.

Diagnostic Tests for Colorectal Cancer

Your doctor will likely perform a variety of diagnostic tests to help confirm or rule out colorectal cancer.

Digital Rectal Exam and Fecal Occult Blood Testing

One of the most important, yet simplest, first-line tests used to screen for colorectal cancer is the *digital rectal examination* or *DRE.* The test is performed at the doctor's office and takes only a few minutes. The doctor inserts a lubricated, gloved finger into the rectum and feels for abnormal areas. The DRE can alert him or her to the presence of rectal tumors. The test should be started at age 40 and be continued every year for life.

During the DRE, your doctor will test your stool for *fecal occult blood (FOB),* which may not be visible to the naked eye. FOB is the main screening test for finding colorectal cancers in the average individual starting at age 50. FOB screening involves placing a smear of stool on a *guaiac card* and mixing it with a drop of a liquid chemical. If a trace amount of blood is present in your stool, the card turns blue, a positive test result. Only 2 to 4 percent of patients tested will be found to have a positive test for fecal occult blood.

A positive FOB test result does *not* necessarily mean you have colorectal cancer. It means your doctor needs to perform additional tests to find the source of the blood. One negative aspect of the fecal occult blood test is its accuracy. The test is not very specific for the presence of colorectal cancer. There are many other diseases of the colon, including hemorrhoids, rectal ulcers, fissures, Crohn's disease, ulcerative colitis, diverticulosis, polyps, and trauma from the exam itself that can cause you to have a positive test result. Despite not being very specific, the fecal occult blood test is simple, cost-effective, and helpful in beginning the process of detecting colorectal cancer.

Blood Tests

Your doctor may order blood tests if he or she suspects the presence of a colorectal cancer. A *complete blood count (CBC)* is a test performed to evaluate your red blood cell count. This test specifically reports on your *hemoglobin* and *hematocrit,* two values necessary to determine your blood count. Hemoglobin is related to the amount of iron circulating in your blood. Hematocrit reports the percentage of red blood cells in your total blood volume. If both values are lower than normal, it's called anemia. Having anemia does not necessarily mean you have colorectal cancer. Anemia can be caused by a number of other health problems. Anemia can also be caused by slowly losing blood over several months from a growing colorectal cancer. If the anemia gets severe, fatigue can set in. The results of your CBC will let your doctor know if you have anemia.

Other blood tests are used to evaluate how well your liver is working and if a suspected colorectal cancer has spread to it. The *liver enzymes* test includes measuring blood levels of *alkaline phosphatase, bilirubin, SGOT, albumin,* and *SGPT*. All these enzymes exist in normal levels in the blood. However, if you have been diagnosed with colorectal cancer and your liver enzymes are high, it may mean the cancer has spread to your liver. Or it may not. Other health problems may cause your liver enzymes to be elevated. Ask your doctor about your liver enzyme test results.

Another blood test used to check for the presence of a colorectal cancer is called the *carcinoembryonic antigen level* or *CEA*. This blood test measures a protein circulating in the blood that can be elevated if a colorectal cancer is present. It is more specific for colorectal cancer than other blood tests because the CEA protein is actually produced by cancer cells. While this test is more specific, it's not perfect. The CEA level can also be elevated due to other types of cancer such as breast, lung, and pancreatic. Ulcerative colitis, chronic lung or liver disease, and cigarette smoking can also elevate CEA levels.

If you've been diagnosed with colorectal cancer and your CEA level is very high, it may indicate the cancer has spread to other organs. When cancer spreads beyond its site of origin, it is called *metastasis*. Some doctors test CEA level before treating colorectal cancer to use the measure as a baseline. More commonly, doctors test CEA after treatment and during follow-up to see how well the treatment is working.

A word of caution about blood tests: If you have abnormal blood test results, *don't panic*. Abnormal test results alone do *not* mean you have colorectal cancer. Your doctor will need to put these results in perspective with your symptoms and the results of your physical examination. Abnormal blood tests will direct your doctor to pursue further testing in order to make a definitive diagnosis.

The next step in diagnosing a colorectal cancer involves more invasive procedures that allow the doctor to see inside your colon. At this point, your family doctor may refer you to a gastroenterologist, a specialist in diseases of the GI tract, or a general surgeon for these tests.

Proctoscopy

A *proctoscope* is a short rigid scope, about a foot in length, that allows your doctor to examine the rectum, the lower-most part of the colon. Called a *proctoscopy*, the procedure may be done in your doctor's office, and may be used if cancer of the rectum is suspected. However, a proctoscope is not used in screening for colorectal cancer, and patients should not consider it as such. In fact, this procedure is rarely used nowadays; most doctors proceed right to the flexible sigmoidoscopy for cancer screening. A proctoscopy is usually done to evaluate such things as bleeding hemorrhoids, which are usually located around or just inside the anus.

Flexible Sigmoidoscopy

One invasive test frequently used to evaluate the inside of the lower part of the colon is the *flexible sigmoidoscopy*. A flexible sigmoidoscope is a thin, flexible fiber-optic tube about thirty inches in length. This tube can be connected to a television monitor in order to magnify what the doctor is seeing. The scope is also made so the doctor can look directly into the end of it and see the inside of the colon as the tube is being advanced. This flexible device allows your doctor to directly examine the last several feet of the colon (sigmoid colon) and the entire rectum. The procedure is carried out in the doctor's office and takes about ten minutes. No anesthesia is necessary since the procedure isn't painful. The procedure may be performed by your primary care doctor, an internist, a gastroenterologist, or general surgeon.

During sigmoidoscopy, the scope is inserted into the anus and directed into the rectum, up to the lower part of the colon. You'll feel a slight pressure sensation as air is pumped through the scope and into the colon. This distends the inside of the colon and rectum so the doctor can examine the entire lining. If a tumor or polyp is discovered, it can be removed for laboratory examination (biopsied) through the sigmoidoscope.

I try to comfort and reassure patients about their upcoming colonoscopy. They are nervous going in. However, once it is all over they often realize that it was not bad at all.

Chris, 41
Nurse

If your doctor orders a sigmoidoscopy, you'll need to do some preparation the day before. You'll be instructed to give yourself an enema the night before the procedure to clean out your rectum. Avoid food/beverages on the morning of the procedure; however, it is okay to take medications with water.

The biggest advantage of flexible sigmoidoscopy is that it enables the doctor to check for polyps or cancer in the lower part of the colon. Nearly 50 percent of all colorectal cancers occur in this area. The disadvantage is, the rest of the colon is beyond the sigmoidoscope's reach, so it can miss precancerous polyps and cancers in other locations. Studies have shown that if your screening flexible sigmoidoscopy is normal, there is up to a 3 percent chance you have a cancer in the other side of your colon, not reached by the sigmoidoscope. This drawback can be eliminated by combining the sigmoidoscopy with other tests such as the double-contrast barium enema.

Possible complications of sigmoidoscopy include perforation of the colon or rectum by the scope. This is rare, occurring in only 1 out of 10,000 procedures. However, if it does occur, emergency surgery is needed to repair the perforation.

Double-Contrast Barium Enema

If your doctor decides your entire colon needs evaluation, he or she may order a *double-contrast barium enema*. This procedure is done in concert with a flexible sigmoidoscopy. The double-contrast barium enema takes an hour and is performed on an outpatient basis in the radiology department of a hospital or surgery center. It is given by a *radiologist*, a doctor trained to perform and read X-rays.

If your doctor orders this test, you will be given advance instructions. The day before the procedure, you will be asked to drink a substance that cleans the inside of your colon.

During the procedure, a rubber tube is placed just inside your rectum. An X-ray liquid (barium) and air are injected into your colon. Several X-ray pictures of your outlined colon are taken. While this test isn't painful, most people experience a sensation of pressure that may be uncomfortable.

Double-contrast barium is accurate enough to identify most large polyps and cancerous colorectal tumors. However, it can miss small polyps less than one inch in size.

Colonoscopy

If a tumor is found, you'll need a *colonoscopy*. Colonoscopy is the most effective way to evaluate the inside of your entire colon for the presence of colorectal cancer. Performed in an

Proctoscopy　　　　**Sigmoidoscopy**　　　　**Colonoscopy**

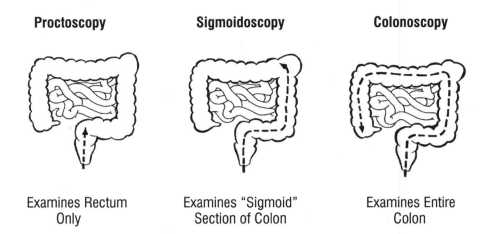

Examines Rectum　　　Examines "Sigmoid"　　　Examines Entire
Only　　　　　　　　Section of Colon　　　　　　Colon

outpatient setting at a hospital or surgery center, it is carried out by either a gastroenterologist or a general surgeon.

The procedure involves gradually advancing a flexible fiber-optic telescope attached to a television monitor through the entire colon. The colonoscope is similar to the flexible sigmoidoscope, though it's several feet longer. It allows the doctor performing the procedure to directly see the inner lining of the entire colon. When performed successfully, colonoscopy is accurate at finding polyps and cancers of all sizes.

Like flexible sigmoidoscopy, a colonoscopy requires preparation. Your colon must be empty and clean before the procedure. This usually involves drinking a purging liquid (Go-Lytely, Fleet phosphosoda, magnesium citrate) a day or two before the procedure. In addition, you'll need to drink only liquids and avoid solid foods one to two days before the procedure. While this preparation to clean out the colon is necessary, it will keep you close to a bathroom. It may be wise to take off from work the day before and the day of the procedure.

When you arrive at the hospital, an intravenous (IV) line will be started so medication can be given during the procedure. You will then be taken to a special room, placed on your side with your knees bent, and given medicine such as Demerol, Versed, morphine, or Valium to sedate you. Sedation is necessary because the procedure can cause some discomforting pressure as the colonoscope is guided through the colon. The pressure is air being pumped into your colon in order to distend it enough so the doctor can see the entire inner lining. The entire procedure takes approximately thirty minutes.

Afterward, you'll be taken to a recovery area and monitored by nurses until the medicine has worn off. You'll need to have someone take you to the procedure and pick you up afterward. Before you leave, ask your doctor to explain what he or she found during the colonoscopy. Normally, if a polyp or tumor is found, your doctor will take pictures. Ask to see these pictures and ask for an explanation. Your doctor may even give you a copy of the pictures if you ask. Upon discharge, you can resume a normal diet and a normal activity schedule.

A variation that is equally effective but less invasive is *virtual colonoscopy*. This procedure requires colon cleansing similar to standard colonoscopy. However, with virtual colonoscopy, a fiber-optic scope is not inserted into the rectum. Instead, you are placed inside a sophisticated computerized tomography (CT or CAT) scanner and instructed to lie still. A computer scans the inside of your colon, generating detailed images. The images are similar to what your doctor sees when he or she performs a regular colonoscopy. Virtual colonoscopy has the advantages of being less physically invasive and less uncomfortable. However, if a polyp is found on a virtual colonoscopy, you will still need a standard colonoscopy to remove it.

Colonoscopy is the most effective way to evaluate your entire colon for polyps and colorectal cancer. It is more comprehensive than a flexible sigmoidoscopy and more accurate than a double-contrast barium enema. If a tumor is found during a colonoscopy, it can be biopsied or even removed through the colonoscope with the assistance of various snare wires and biopsy forceps.

The main disadvantage of a colonoscopy is possible complications, including bleeding after polyp removal and perforation of the colon. Perforation doesn't occur often (0.2 to 0.4 percent of the time), but it requires emergency surgery to repair. In addition, a colonoscopy requires intravenous sedation that may cause adverse reactions.

Failure to visualize the entire colon is also a possible problem with colonoscopy. Sometimes—10 to 20 percent of the time—it's impossible for the doctor to navigate all the tortuous turns in the colon and see the right side. When this occurs, a follow-up barium enema is necessary to complete the examination.

Colonoscopy is also more expensive than other diagnostic tests. Colonoscopy costs $750 to $2,000 compared with $100 to $300 for flexible sigmoidoscopy and $10 to $20 for fecal occult blood (FOB) testing.

Other Diagnostic Tests

Your doctor may order other tests if he or she suspects colorectal cancer. Many times these tests are ordered to evaluate if a newly diagnosed cancer has spread to other parts of the body. They are also ordered in anticipation of treatment, such as surgery or chemotherapy. All are carried out in an outpatient setting, involve no discomfort, and help fill in pieces of the diagnostic puzzle for the doctor.

X-rays

An X-ray of your chest is a helpful screening tool to rule out any underlying lung disease and potential cancer spread to the lungs. A chest X-ray is usually ordered before surgery once a colorectal cancer is diagnosed. Plain X-rays of your abdomen can also be done to make sure a colorectal cancer is not blocking your intestine. X-rays of your bones can also be done to evaluate whether a newly diagnosed cancer has spread.

Computerized Axial Tomography Scan

A *computerized axial tomography (CT* or *CAT) scan* of the abdomen and pelvis is sometimes ordered to look at a cross section of all the organs inside the abdominal cavity. The test involves drinking a bitter-tasting liquid, called *contrast*, several hours before the procedure. This liquid migrates into your colon over several hours so it can be seen during the X-rays. You may also be given intravenous contrast during the test to further enhance the images seen on film.

Once the contrast is in place, you will be taken to the X-ray department and asked to lie still in a large doughnut-shaped scanner. While lying in the scanner, a technician will periodically ask you to take deep breaths and hold them as the X-rays are taken. The pictures from the CT are very detailed cross-sectional views of all the organs in your abdominal cavity.

The CT test takes about thirty minutes and is performed on an outpatient basis. It is often carried out before surgery to evaluate for the spread of a colorectal cancer to other organs, specifically the liver. If a suspicious spot is seen in the liver, a radiologist can use the CT scan to guide a needle to it and obtain a biopsy. If a cancer of the rectum is suspected, the radiologist may place some X-ray liquid inside your rectum during the procedure. This liquid, called *rectal contrast,* enhances visualization of the cancer.

Magnetic Resonance Imaging (MRI)

An *MRI scan* may be performed in patients with colorectal cancer. It can evaluate if the cancer has spread to other organs in the body. Unlike CT scans and most X-rays, MRI does not use a radioactive energy source to generate very detailed pictures of internal organs. The test doesn't require any liquid X-ray prep. It is also more specific than a CT for evaluating brain or spinal cord involvement.

One disadvantage is that most MRI scanners are closed spaces, requiring patients to lie on a table and pass through a tube, where the images are recorded. This may cause claustrophobia in some people. Often doctors order sedative medicine for patients to calm fears. Some hospitals now offer "open" MRI machines, which have larger openings for the patient to pass through.

Ultrasound

Ultrasound tests of the abdominal organs, specifically the liver, can also be used to evaluate for the spread of colorectal cancer. An ultrasound may be used as a screening test before a CT scan. Ultrasound is less expensive, but it is not as accurate as a CT scan and the quality of ultrasound pictures depends on the expertise of the technician performing the test.

Transrectal ultrasound involves placing a thin probe inside the rectum adjacent to a newly discovered cancer. The sound waves penetrate the tumor and can give information about how deeply the cancer has invaded the rectal wall or its spread to other organs. This information is important for surgical treatment.

Bone Scan

Your doctor may also use a bone scan to test for the spread of a colorectal cancer. The bone scan evaluates all the bones in your skeleton for evidence of tumor spread. Colorectal cancer can spread to any bone in the body. If you have just been diagnosed with a colorectal cancer and have a new pain in your shoulder or back, let your doctor know.

Bone scans are performed in an outpatient setting in the nuclear medicine section of the radiology department. While a bone scan involves the injection of X-ray material, the test is not painful. The X-ray material will become concentrated in your bones, and pictures will be taken as you lie still in a large scanner.

Cystogram

Used to determine whether cancer has spread into the bladder, this test involves a dye being injected into the bladder through the urethra. Then, X-rays are taken; the dye helps with the identification of any abnormal growths in the bladder.

Referrals to Specialists

Depending on your condition, your family doctor may refer you to specialists who can help with the diagnosis and treatment of your colorectal cancer. These specialists may include *gastroenterologists, general surgeons,* and *colorectal surgeons.*

Gastroenterologists are doctors trained in internal medicine who go on to a two-year fellowship, specializing in the field of gastroenterology, diagnosing and treating diseases of the colon. Gastroenterologists receive special training in how to perform diagnostic procedures to look inside the colon. Once a gastroenterologist examines you and makes a definitive diagnosis of colorectal cancer, he or she will refer you to a surgeon for treatment.

Both general and colorectal surgeons are trained to perform procedures on the colon and to surgically treat colorectal cancer. Colorectal surgeons are trained in general surgery for at least five years. After this, they obtain specialized training by doing a colorectal fellowship.

Questions to Ask Your Doctor

- When should I start to get screened and how often?
- Which screening test is best for me?
- If a tumor or polyp was found on colonoscopy, did you biopsy or remove it?
- Where in my colon was this tumor or polyp found?
- What other tests will I need to have done to make sure the cancer has not spread?

4

Coping Emotionally

Nothing can prepare you for a diagnosis of cancer. With it comes a flood of stressful emotions—shock, disbelief, anger, depression, hopelessness, fear, denial. At first, it may be difficult to comprehend that you have cancer. Many people feel the diagnosis just "comes out of nowhere" and "knocks the emotional wind out of you." Especially in the beginning, when things just seem to be happening too fast, you may feel as if you are losing control. It's a very troubling and stressful time for the whole family.

Shock and disbelief are especially common reactions to the diagnosis of colorectal cancer because many people have no warning signs. Patients often say, "How could this be happening to me? I feel fine. I had no clue." Colorectal cancer is commonly discovered during routine examinations and blood tests in patients who are otherwise feeling well. Some people actually deny the reality of their disease, refusing to accept the diagnosis. "This isn't happening to me. It's impossible." If they persist in denying the reality of their colorectal cancer, it can interfere with their treatment and survival.

Fear is another emotion colorectal cancer patients and their loved ones face. They're afraid of what lies ahead. They're afraid because they don't know if the cancer has spread. They fear having to wear a colostomy, an external sack for waste removal. (Most patients today do *not* need a colostomy.) They fear becoming a burden on their families. Most commonly, they fear dying because we associate the word cancer with death.

You may also feel hopeless about your condition. The word *cancer* traditionally isn't associated with hope. However, there is plenty to be hopeful about. Today, the cure rate for colorectal cancer diagnosed and treated early is 90 percent. New and more effective treatments are being developed every day. In addition, dozens of cancer survivor groups can provide you with valuable information and emotional support.

All your feelings and reactions are normal and under-standable. However, it's important to recognize and cope with your feelings because negative emotions can be very detrimental to your health. Anxiety and stress can lead to lack of sleep, poor appetite, weight loss, poor judgment, and make you physically sick. Research has shown that stress like that caused by negative emotions can depress the immune system and make recovery more difficult. With help from your loved ones and your doctors, it's possible to gain some perspective on your feelings and focus on the positive factors that can help you beat colorectal cancer.

Support from Friends and Family

During this difficult time, it's the people closest to you who will be your best supporters. Do not be afraid to lean on or open up to them. They want to help. Often people can help by listening or just being there.

Here are some tips for getting the support you need and coping with the emotional side of your condition:

Assemble your support team. Think about who is closest to you—friends, family, co-workers. Who do you feel comfortable talking with? Who might be available to help you with practical matters like driving you to doctor visits? Make a list of people you'd like on your support team. Then ask them if they'll be available for you during this difficult time.

Talk about how you feel. Tell your spouse/partner, family, friends, and other members of your support team about your anxieties and fears. Don't try to "protect" your loved ones by keeping your feelings bottled up inside. It helps to get your feelings out in the open. Let them talk about their fears, too.

Don't be shy. Cancer is difficult to talk about. This is especially true of colorectal cancers. People shy away from talking about anything affecting their bowels. Friends, family, and coworkers may find it awkward in the beginning to talk about your condition because of their own anxieties and fears. Talking about your colorectal cancer will help remove the stigma.

Avoid blaming yourself. It's nobody's "fault" that you have colorectal cancer. Avoid playing the "blame game" and concentrate on getting better.

Let others know what you need. Maybe you need someone to talk with, someone to take care of the children, or a ride to the doctor's office. Let your friends and family know how they can support you.

Look for the positive. Focus on the fact that the cancer was diagnosed early and there is a very good chance of being cured. Or concentrate on the fact that new and better treatments are being developed every day. Staying positive won't guarantee you'll beat the disease, but it'll make it easier to cope.

Getting Professional/Community Support

Sometimes the emotional burden of a cancer diagnosis is so overwhelming you need more support than your family and friends can provide. Don't hesitate to seek professional help in dealing with your emotions. Many professional counselors specialize in helping people cope with cancer. Ask your doctor or the social service department at the hospital for referrals to mental health therapists in your community.

Denial is a pretty normal initial reaction to a cancer diagnosis. By overcoming the denial, patients can become more involved in understanding their disease and its treatment.

Becky
Nurse

Sometimes it also helps to talk with others who have "been there." Other cancer survivors can provide emotional support, practical information, and advice. There are a number of cancer survivor support groups available. Cancer support meetings are helpful in sorting out the emotions and fears that come with the diagnosis of cancer. They can also put you in touch with others who have had a similar cancer who can share their experiences. One or more of these people can become your buddies, providing mutual support and comfort. Ask your doctor about these support groups or call the local chapter of the American Cancer Society for referrals to groups in your community.

Your health-care professionals, including your doctors, can be a tremendous source of information and support for you. If you feel overwhelmed by your emotions, don't be afraid to talk with your doctor. Tell him or her how you feel. Often, having your doctor tell you that your feelings are normal and very common can ease fears and anxieties. Many times fears are unfounded and can be replaced with information your doctor can provide.

Here are some tips for working with your doctors and other health-care professionals to cope with your feelings:

Tell your doctor about your feelings. Don't be embarrassed or try to hide your fears and anxieties.

Ask for help. If you're having difficulty coping with your feelings, ask your doctor for a referral to a mental health professional.

Ask questions. Don't be afraid to ask questions about your diagnosis, treatment options, and prognosis. If your doctor uses terms you don't understand, ask him or her to explain in simpler terms or draw you a picture. Keep asking until you understand.

Learn all you can. Knowledge is power. It can put you in control of your emotions and help you make informed decisions about your treatment. Talk with all your doctors. Ask them for printed materials about your condition. Seek out information in books, on the Internet, and from talking with other cancer survivors.

5

Staging Colorectal Cancer

taging a newly discovered cancer is the process of determining how far the cancer has spread at the time of diagnosis. It involves putting together all the test results, X-rays, and, once the cancer has been removed, the final tissue report produced by a pathologist. Once all the information has been gathered and analyzed, your doctor will place your cancer in a category, or stage. Staging your colorectal cancer is critical in determining what type of treatment you will receive, your chances of being cured, and your long-term prognosis. The stage of your disease at the time of diagnosis will determine whether your treatment involves surgery alone or a combination of surgery with chemotherapy and/or radiation. Staging is also important in understanding how soon and where in the body a cancer may recur during your lifetime.

To understand the staging process, let's review how a colorectal cancer grows and spreads. As mentioned earlier, a cancer starts to grow from the inner lining of the colon (mucosa). It grows from the inside out, through the middle layer (muscle) and ultimately through the outermost layer (serosa).

If the cancer extends through the entire colon wall, it can involve the adjacent lymph nodes. These glands filter the blood for infectious organisms as part of your immune system. With cancer, lymph nodes act as the first barrier to cancer cell spread. There are hundreds of lymph nodes throughout your body. They are visible to the naked eye, oval in shape, and normally the size of a raisin when not inflamed or involved with cancer. You may notice that when you have a sore throat, the lymph nodes in your neck become enlarged because of the infection. In people with colorectal cancer, the lymph nodes adjacent to the tumor can be involved with cancer cells.

Once cancer cells get into the lymph nodes, tumor cells can escape into the bloodstream and go anywhere the blood goes. Beyond the lymph nodes, the liver is the most common site for cancer spread. This occurs because the blood supply from the entire colon drains into the liver first. Any tumor cells in the blood leaving the colon will first become lodged in the liver. Colorectal cancer can also spread to the lungs, bones, bladder, brain, ovaries, and *peritoneum,* the thin lining surrounding all the abdominal organs. Below is a list of organs in the body where colorectal cancer can spread and the tests doctors use to document it.

Before your doctor can fully stage your colorectal cancer, he or she needs to answer the following questions.

- What is the extent of tumor growth through the colon wall?
- Are the lymph nodes near the cancer involved with tumor?
- Has the cancer spread to other organs?

The answers to the first two questions can only be obtained after you are surgically treated and have the cancerous segment and lymph nodes removed. If your doctor suspects the cancer has spread, he or she may perform some of the X-ray and blood tests discussed earlier. However, if all the tests are negative, determining if the cancer has spread to other organs will have to be answered at the time of surgery.

Pathology Report

After surgery, a *pathologist* will look under the microscope at all the tissue removed. He or she will then determine how far the cancer has spread through the colorectal wall and if the lymph nodes are involved. A pathologist is a doctor trained to examine tissue and organs for disease. It usually takes two to four days after surgery to obtain a final pathology report. The report should be on your medical chart before you are discharged from the hospital.

The earlier you find a growing cancer, the earlier the stage. This scenario leads to the best chance for a cure.

Kyle
Surgeon

The pathology report will determine your cancer stage. The stage, in turn, will determine if you need further treatment, your long-term prognosis, and the chances of the cancer coming back. The pathology report will include the dimensions/weight of the specimen removed and the important staging information listed below.

Type of Cancer Cells Present

Adenocarcinoma: invasive cancer cells arising from the normal cells lining the colon. The most common type of colorectal cancer seen.

Carcinoma in situ: cells that display very early cancerous changes with a very low capability to spread if treated early.

Dysplasia: precancerous changes observed in normal cells.

Degree of Differentiation

The report will describe the degree of genetic chaos inside the cancer cells as seen under the microscope. There are three degrees of differentiation: poorly, moderately, and well differentiated. Poorly differentiated cells are very chaotic, more aggressive than the other two types, and have the worst prognosis. Well-differentiated cancer cells are not that aggressive and have the best prognosis.

Spread to Blood Vessels

Known as *extramural venous invasion*, this condition means the cancer cells have invaded the walls of the small blood vessels surrounding the tumor and have the potential to leak into the bloodstream. This is not a favorable characteristic, as it increases the risk of spread to other organs in the body.

Colorectal Cancer Spread Sites and Diagnostic Tests

Body Site	Tests
Liver	CT Scan, MRI, Ultrasound
Ovaries	Ultrasound, CT Scan
Lungs	Chest X-ray, CT Scan, MRI
Bones	Bone Scan
Bladder, Small Intestine	CT Scan, Cystogram
Brain, Spine	CT Scan, MRI

Resection Margins

Resection margins are the ends of the colorectal specimen removed. (*Resection* means "removal of.") The pathologist will analyze them for evidence of cancer cells. If the resection margins are free of tumor, then no further treatment is needed. If the resection margins contain cancer cells, this is less favorable and requires further treatment.

Extent of Tumor Growth

This part of the report describes how far the cancer has grown into the colorectal wall. The best-case scenario has the tumor confined to the inner layer. The worst-case scenario has the tumor growing through all the layers and invading the *pericolonic fat*. In such a case, the chances are high for recurrence of the cancer. In addition, the further a cancer grows through the colorectal wall, the greater the chance of it spreading to the lymph nodes.

Lymph Node Involvement

The report will list the lymph nodes as being positive or negative for cancer. Negative means no cancerous cells were found in the lymph nodes. Positive lymph node involvement indicates lymph nodes were found to have cancer cells. Positive lymph nodes decrease overall survival and mean further treatment will be needed. In addition, the number of lymph nodes involved is also important toward prognosis. A worse prognosis is observed if more than four lymph nodes are involved.

Stages of Colorectal Cancer

Once the doctor determines the TNM classification for your cancer, he or she will be able to place you in one of four stages.

Stage I

This stage means the cancer is confined to the inner layer of the colon wall, does not involve the lymph nodes, and has not spread to other organs. Stage I describes an early colorectal cancer and has the best prognosis. Ninety percent of people with this stage are alive five years after initial treatment.

Stage II

This stage describes a cancer that has grown through the entire colon wall. However, there is no evidence of lymph node involvement or spread to other organs. In this stage, 60 to 80 percent of patients are alive five years after their initial treatment. About 40 percent of all patients diagnosed have stage I or II cancer.

Prior to my operation, my surgeon was very good at explaining the stages of colon cancer and how it can grow.

Peggy, 56
Survivor

Stage III

This stage describes a colorectal cancer that involves any part of the colon wall and the lymph nodes as well. When the lymph nodes are involved with cancer, further treatment is usually needed after surgery. In this stage, 40 to 60 percent of patients are alive five years after their initial treatment. About 35 percent of all patients diagnosed are determined to have a stage III cancer.

Stage IV

When a colorectal cancer is stage IV, it means it has spread beyond the colon wall to other organs, such as the liver or lungs. This stage requires further treatment after surgery and has the worst prognosis. Only 5 percent of patients with stage IV are alive five years after their initial treatment. About 10 to 15 percent of all patients are diagnosed with an advanced, stage IV cancer.

Stages of Tumor Growth in Colon Wall

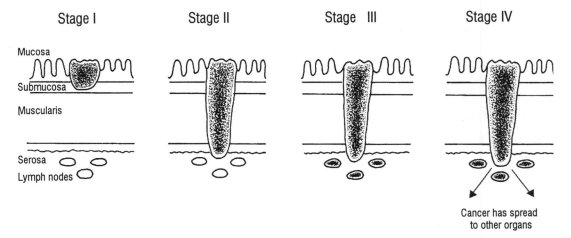

Cancer has spread to other organs

TNM Staging System

To record the extent of any spread of the cancer or lymph node involvement, pathologists use the TNM classification system. It is a universal staging system adopted by the American Joint Committee on Cancer (AJCC). This system uses three letters—T, N, M—to describe the extent of a cancer.

The letter **T** is used to describe the extent of tumor growth into the colon wall. T is given a number (1-4), depending on how far into the colon wall the tumor has grown.

The letter **N** is used to describe whether the lymph nodes are involved. If lymph nodes are not involved, your cancer is designated N-0. If the lymph nodes are involved, your cancer is designated N-1.

The letter **M** describes whether the cancer has spread to other organs. If there is no evidence of spread, then M-0 is the designation. If there is evidence of spread to other organs, the designation is M-1.

For a complete description of the TNM classification system and other staging systems, see the appendix of this book.

Questions to Ask Your Doctor

- What is the stage of my cancer?
- Is my cancer confined to my colon, or has it spread?
- Are the lymph nodes involved?
- Based on my stage, what is my five-year survival?
- Based on my stage, what are the chances of my cancer coming back within the first two years after treatment?

Patients never meet me, however, my job is vital in determining how far their cancer has grown into the colon wall and determining the stage of their cancer.

Frank
Pathologist

6

Surgery

After your colorectal cancer has been diagnosed and all the X-ray tests are complete, the next step is to formulate a treatment plan. The first line of treatment is surgery if tests indicate the cancer has not spread to other organs, which is true for approximately 75 percent of cases. If it has been determined the cancer has already spread to other organs, then an operation may not be the first line of treatment.

For most newly diagnosed colorectal cancer patients, surgery is the primary treatment and offers the best chance for a cure. An operation for colorectal cancer is major surgery, involving general anesthesia. The goal of any operation for colorectal cancer is to remove the portion of the colon that contains the growing cancer, along with the surrounding lymph nodes, and to reconnect the two ends.

Who Performs Colorectal Cancer Surgery?

After you've been diagnosed, your doctor will refer you to a surgeon for treatment. This will either be a general surgeon or a colorectal surgeon. Both are equally trained and qualified to perform surgery on the colon for cancer. A general surgeon has completed at least five years of surgical training, much of that involving operations on the gastrointestinal tract. A colorectal surgeon has also completed at least five years of training in general surgery and an additional one to two years of specialty training in diseases of the colon. Both should be board certified in surgery and perform operations on the colon regularly.

Operations for Colon Cancer

Polypectomy

Polypectomy is the surgical removal of a polyp. This is often performed by a gastroenterologist or surgeon during a colonoscopy. In this procedure, the doctor uses an assortment of wires, snares, and small forceps to remove a polyp through the colonoscope while you are sedated. Most polyps that are under one inch in diameter and growing on a stalk, like a mushroom, can be removed this way. However, polyps larger than one inch in diameter, broad based, or containing cancer cells require an operation to remove a part of the colon and the surrounding lymph nodes.

Partial Colectomy

Partial colectomy is the removal of part of the colon. It is the most common type of operation performed for colon cancer. Partial colectomy is major surgery. It involves the surgeon making a six- to twelve-inch vertical incision in the middle of your abdomen. The operation takes one to three hours and involves a five- to seven-day recovery in the hospital.

When a partial colectomy is carried out, only the portion of the colon with the cancer inside is removed. This is like removing a broken link in a chain and reconnecting the rest of the good links. Once the cancerous segment is removed, the two free ends of colon are reattached. Surgeons can sew both ends together with a suture or metal staples. If a suture is used, your body will absorb it over several months. If metal staples are used, they are left in place permanently. Both techniques are equally effective. Surgeons have individual preferences.

The type of partial colectomy you may need depends on where the tumor is located. If the cancer is located in the right colon, the operation performed is called a right colectomy since only the right part of the colon is removed. To remove a cancer in the transverse colon, a transverse colectomy is needed. A cancer located in the left colon is removed by a left colectomy. One located in the sigmoid colon is removed by a sigmoid colectomy.

The goal of all partial colectomies is to remove the colon segment with the cancer neatly tucked away inside. Surgeons cannot just open up the colon and scoop out the cancer. This could cause cancer cells to break loose, enter the bloodstream, and go to other organs in the body. It would also expose other organs to infection by releasing the bacteria normally living inside the colon.

Another goal of partial colectomy is to have at least six inches of normal colon tissue surrounding either side of the cancer after it is removed. This six inches of normal colon tissue is called the margin. An adequate margin of normal colon tissue is necessary to minimize the risk of the cancer coming back in the same area after the two free ends are reconnected.

Subtotal and Total Colectomy

Subtotal colectomy removes more than 90 percent of the colon. It's not a common operation. However, it may be necessary when a person has two separate colon cancers in two different parts of the colon. During this major abdominal operation, the surgeon is still able to reattach both ends of normal colon once the two cancerous segments are removed.

Total colectomy removes the entire colon. Again, this is not a common operation for colon cancer. It is generally performed for other diseases of the colon. It takes about three hours and involves a seven-day recovery in the hospital.

Operations for Rectal Cancer

Polypectomy

A rectal polyp can also be removed through the colonoscope at the time of a colonoscopy. Most polyps found in the rectum can be removed this way. However, rectal polyps greater than one inch and with a broad base may be difficult to remove without a larger operation. In addition, polyps found to have cancer in them once removed by the colonoscope may require more extensive surgery.

Transanal Excision

Transanal excision of a polyp or early cancer in the rectum involves surgical removal through the anus. This is a unique approach since most operations for colorectal cancer involve making a six- to twelve-inch vertical incision through the middle of the abdomen. By oper- ating through the anus and not the abdominal cavity, there is much less trauma to the body and less physical pain. This approach is appropriate if you have a polyp just inside the anus that is not cancerous and cannot be removed at the time of colonoscopy.

If you have a small polyp with some early cancerous cells present just inside the anus, the transanal approach might be appropriate and can save you from undergoing a much larger operation. However, additional treatment such as radiation may be needed to kill any potential cancer cells left behind. The operation is carried out under general anesthesia in the operating room and can take one hour. It can be performed in an outpatient setting. Some patients may need to stay overnight in the hospital.

Low Anterior Resection

A *low anterior resection* removes a cancer located in the lower one-third of the sigmoid colon or upper two-thirds of the rectum. This major operation is very effective. It involves general anesthesia and takes approximately two hours. During the procedure, the surgeon makes a vertical incision starting above the belly button and removes about a twelve-inch portion of the sigmoid colon and rectum. The adjacent lymph nodes are also removed. After removing the cancerous segment, the surgeon reattaches the two free ends together so normal bowel movements can occur. Recovery in the hospital takes at least seven days.

Anterior-Posterior Resection

Anterior-posterior resection, or *AP resection*, is performed on rectal cancers located just inside the anus. The operation takes three hours, requires general anesthesia, and involves a twelve-inch vertical incision on your abdomen.

When a cancer is located less than six to twelve inches from the outside of the anus, this operation may offer the best chance for a cure. If the surgeon can feel the cancer on rectal examination, then chances are an anterior-posterior resection is the necessary operation. It involves removing the segment of rectum housing the cancer, the surrounding lymph nodes, and the anus. It is necessary to remove the anus to make sure the entire cancer is removed. When this is done your surgeon will need to sew up the skin where your anus was. Technically, this procedure of surgically bringing the open end of the colon through the abdominal wall and sewing it to the skin is called a *colostomy*. (*Ostomy* means "opening.") The portion of the open colon brought to the skin is called the *stoma*.

Colostomy also refers to an external plastic bag attached to the skin when surgery requires the closure of the anus. Fecal matter passes through an opening and into the bag. Self-care with a permanent colostomy is covered in detail in chapter 10.

Surgery to treat colorectal cancer is the best chance patients have to be cured if the cancer is caught early. It is major surgery, however, most patients recover completely to live normal, active lives.

Robert Surgeon

Pelvic Exenteration

Pelvic exenteration is to be considered when a cancer of the rectum has invaded nearby organs such as the urinary bladder, uterus, or ovaries. In this situation, the best chance for curing a patient is to remove all the organs attached to the rectal cancer at once, without disturbing any cancer cells. This major operation is seldom performed today.

Colostomy: Temporary or Permanent?

Once they find out they need surgery, many patients worry about needing a *permanent colostomy*. Normally this is *not* the case. According to the National Cancer Institute, only about 15

Surgeries for Colorectal Cancer

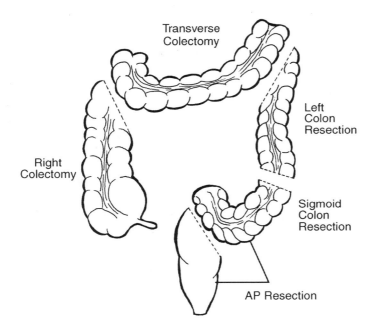

Transverse Colectomy

Left Colon Resection

Right Colectomy

Sigmoid Colon Resection

AP Resection

percent of people with colorectal cancer require a permanent colostomy. The type of operation you need depends on the location of the cancer. Once this has been determined by the diagnostic tests already mentioned, your surgeon will talk with you about the specifics of your operation.

A permanent colostomy will be required if the surgeon has no free end of colon or rectum to go back in and reconnect to. Accordingly, if the cancer is located in the rectum close to the anus, a colostomy may be required to adequately treat the cancer.

In some situations a *temporary colostomy* is required, usually in the case of emergency colon surgery. Why? To avoid infection. Before any planned colorectal operation, the surgeon gives colon-cleansing instructions to follow two days before the surgery. Colon cleansing is necessary so your surgeon can remove the cancerous segment of colon, sew the two remaining ends together, and not worry about infection. When there is no time to clean the colon, as in the case of emergency surgery, the risk of life-threatening infection is very high if the two ends of a "dirty" colon are sewn together after the cancerous segment has been removed. The best way to minimize this risk is to give the patient a colostomy at the time of the operation.

If a patient suffers an acute colonic blockage caused by a growing cancer, emergency surgery and a colostomy are required. Or, if a patient has a cancer that has eroded through and perforated the colon wall, causing feces and bacteria to spill out and creating a life-threatening intra-abdominal infection, emergency surgery to remove the cancerous segment and a colostomy are required.

A temporary colostomy is usually in place four to six months, enough time for everything to heal up inside. The surgeon can then go back in and reconnect the colostomy end to the end left behind in a planned, elective operation. This reversal of the colostomy is called a *colostomy takedown*. This major operation, which takes several hours, involves general anesthesia and a week's recovery in the hospital. Colostomy takedown frees the person of having to wear a plastic pouch and restores normal bowel habits.

After abdominal surgery, the intestines "go to sleep" for 3-5 days. Once the intestines become active, patients will start to pass gas and their doctors can start them on whole foods.

Marie
Nurse

Laparoscopic Surgery

Laparoscopic surgery, also known as *minimally invasive surgery* or *laser surgery*, is being performed more frequently to treat a variety of diseases, including colorectal cancer. Laparoscopic surgery involves smaller incisions and smaller instruments than traditional surgery. Thin, fiber-optic cameras attached to television monitors become the "eyes" of the surgeons as they manipulate small instruments. Smaller incisions mean less pain after surgery, quicker recovery in the hospital, fewer scars, and a shorter time needed to get back to a normal routine.

Laparoscopic operations for colorectal cancer are available in some communities. Medical studies show that patients have less trauma and recover faster with this approach. However, these operations are complex and are more difficult to master than the traditional operations involving larger incisions. Many surgeons today do not have much experience with these operations and are not performing them. In addition, despite being as effective and as safe as traditional surgery, laparoscopic surgery for colorectal cancer is still being studied. Since this approach has been around less than ten years, many surgeons do not feel comfortable performing laparoscopic colorectal cancer surgery until more studies confirm its long-term effectiveness. Ask your surgeon about this type of surgery and its role in treating your disease.

Possible Complications of Colorectal Surgery

The risk for complications after colorectal cancer surgery depends on a number of factors. Your underlying health and existing medical conditions prior to the operation can affect whether you develop complications. If you have high blood pressure, a heart condition, lung disease, or diabetes, you are at a slightly higher risk for developing complications. People who have diabetes and/or who are obese, for instance, are prone to develop wound infections after surgery. If you are healthy prior to surgery, do not smoke, are physically active, and are not overweight, your risk for complications is minimal.

Whether your surgery is planned or performed on an emergency basis impacts your risk for complications, too. An elective, planned operation takes place in a controlled setting under optimum conditions so the risks are small. Emergency surgery has a higher complication rate.

Complications following colorectal surgery are relatively rare, occurring in less than 5 percent of patients. However, the complications can be life threatening if they aren't recognized and treated immediately. Possible complications include heart attack, pneumonia, wound infection, blood clots in the legs (with potential spread to the lungs, causing death), intra-abdominal infection or associated abscess, and *fistula,* an abnormal connection between the intestine and the skin. Fistula occurs when something has punctured the intestine and stool leaks out. It can lead to a serious infection requiring antibiotics. Most fistulas, however, heal spontaneously and do not require surgery. Even in the 5 percent of patients who do experience postsurgical complications, most respond to treatment and do not require further surgery.

Preparation for Colorectal Surgery

There are several things you can do to maximize your chance for a successful operation and minimize your risk for complications.

Ask your surgeon about your daily routines. Do you need to change your eating or exercise habits before surgery?

Stop smoking. Stopping smoking is very important to minimize your risk of lung complications following surgery. Your doctor can provide nicotine patches and refer you to smoking cessation programs to help you quit.

Ask about medications. Which medications do you need to take prior to surgery? Which ones should you stop taking? If you take a blood-thinning medication such as Coumadin, aspirin, or Motrin, stop taking it at least seven days before your surgery. Also, let your doctor know about any herbal preparations or vitamin/mineral supplements you take. Some of them have been associated with complications.

Ask your doctor about taking home an incentive spirometer. This device is effective for improving breathing immediately after surgery. No bigger than a bread-box, it is light and mobile and has a plastic tube that you blow into. Take one home and practice with it one week before your operation.

Carefully follow your bowel prep instructions. Proper bowel prep can minimize infection and maximize the success of your surgery. Your surgeon should provide you with step-by-step instructions. Two days prior to surgery, you'll need to begin a liquid diet as directed by your doctor. The next step involves drinking either a gallon of a lime-flavored purging liquid or several tablespoons of Fleets Phosphosoda mixed with water. In addition, your doctor will give you several antibiotic pills to complete the bowel preparation process.

Consider your own blood. Some people worry about receiving tainted blood in a blood transfusion during or after surgery. All donated blood is rigorously tested, so the risk of receiving tainted blood is very low, less than 0.01 percent. However, to alleviate this concern, you can donate your own blood weeks in advance of the operation or have a relative with the same blood type donate blood for you. By setting up your own (*autologous)* blood or a relative's donated blood, the risk of receiving tainted blood drops to zero. Prior to your operation, ask your surgeon about the chances of requiring a blood transfusion and the feasibility of donating your own blood.

The Day of Your Operation

At the hospital on the morning of your operation, you'll be asked to fill out several admission and registration forms. Next you'll change into a hospital gown and enter the *preoperative holding area,* the last stop before entering the operating room. Loved ones will be able to stay with you in the holding area right up to the time you go into the operating room. Here, you'll meet the nurses and the anesthesiologist who will be involved in your operation. Your surgeon may also come by to see if you have any last-minute questions or concerns.

While you're in the preoperative holding area, an *intravenous (IV) line* will be started in your arm, and your medical chart will be examined for completeness. You will also be given antibiotics through the IV. Just before you enter the operating room, the anesthesiologist will give you an intravenous medicine to ease any nervousness you may have.

In the Operating Room

You'll be brought into the operating room on a gurney and asked to move onto a narrow table. At the head of this table, in the middle of the operating room, are anesthesia machines and monitoring devices used during surgery. The nurses will be busy getting the surgical instruments ready while your surgeon washes his or her hands. The anesthesiologist will inject a milk-like fluid into your intravenous line to put you to sleep. This is general anesthesia, which will render you totally unconscious. You won't be able to feel or hear anything once the drug takes effect.

While you're asleep, the anesthesiologist will place a breathing tube down your throat and into your windpipe (*trachea*). This tube, attached to a machine, will breathe for you during the surgery. A thin, rubber tube called a *catheter* will then be placed by a nurse into your bladder. It monitors the amount of urine your kidneys produce during the operation and is usually left in place for several days after the operation. A final plastic tube, a *nasogastric tube,* will be placed in your throat and advanced into your stomach by the anesthesiologist. It is used to keep your stomach empty during the operation and will be left in place when you wake up from the surgery. Finally, *pneumatic compression stockings* will be placed on both of your legs. The stockings periodically squeeze the calf muscles to prevent blood clots from forming during the operation. Your surgeon will usually order these stockings removed two or three days after your surgery, when you are better able to walk.

During the operation, your surgeon will be cutting and dividing various tissues. He or she will remove the cancerous segment of your colon and reconnect the two free ends together. Your surgeon will also inspect all the other organs in your abdominal cavity to look for evidence that the cancer has spread. If a suspicious nodule or mass is found, especially in the liver, the surgeon will remove a piece for laboratory examination (biopsy). Once the operation is complete, the breathing tube is removed immediately before you completely wake up. Once the anesthesiologist gives the okay, you will be placed back on a gurney and taken to the *recovery room.*

Recovery Room

You will be in the recovery room for the first hour immediately after your surgery. Your vital signs (blood pressure, heart rate, and respiration rate) will be closely monitored and checked by the nurses.

It's after surgery that pain becomes an issue. Be sure to discuss your postoperative pain control options with your surgeon *before* your operation. You will experience some pain after surgery. However, it can be adequately controlled by a number of options. You can be given periodic injections of narcotic drugs. You can be hooked up to a *patient-controlled anesthesia (PCA)* pump that administers a continuous dose of narcotics over a twenty-four-hour period. The PCA pump also allows you to administer additional narcotic booster injections through a handheld device if the pain worsens. The PCA pump provides steadier, more even postoperative pain control than traditional injections. A final method of pain control uses an *epidural catheter.* The catheter is a tiny tube that is inserted in the middle of your back and guided close to your spinal cord. It is placed by an anesthesiologist prior to your going to sleep in the operating room and is left in place for several days after surgery. The catheter allows the anesthesiologist to continuously infuse narcotic pain medicine through a pump at your bedside. This continuous infusion affects the nerves that cause you to feel pain from the surgery. It is a very effective way to control pain after major abdominal operations.

In the recovery room, nurses will administer whatever pain control method your surgeon has ordered. While you're in recovery, your family will be notified of your progress. Once the anesthesiologist is satisfied that your vital signs are stable and you are breathing adequately on your own, he or she will release you to a hospital room.

Recovering in the Hospital

Barring any major complications, most patients need a week in the hospital to recover from major colorectal cancer surgery. Complications may keep you in the hospital longer. The physical stress from the operation causes several things in your body to stop working normally, and it takes a week for these things to get back to normal. During this time, your surgeon will see you every day. He or she will monitor your recovery and decide when to remove tubes, decrease your pain medicine, when you should get out of bed, have your dressing changed, and when to feed you. All these decisions are dependent upon how soon your bodily functions return to normal.

Pain Management

While pain control starts in the recovery room, it continues in the hospital ward. Your postoperative pain should improve with each passing day in the hospital. If you feel your pain is not being adequately controlled, don't be afraid to tell your nurse or your surgeon. Do not just "grin and bear" the pain or think it is part of the normal healing process. You are *not* being a bothersome patient by asking your surgeon to try something else to relieve your pain.

If a PCA pump was started in the recovery room by your surgeon, it will continue working while you're recovering in the ward. If an epidural catheter was placed prior to surgery, it will usually be removed three to four days after surgery. Once you begin to drink liquids or eat solid food, your surgeon will switch your pain medication from intravenous fluid to pills that can be taken by mouth. Most oral pain medication today is a derivative of the narcotic codeine and comes in various strengths. If you are allergic to codeine, talk with your doctor about other pain control medications.

Regaining Bowel Function

The length of your hospital stay depends largely on how long it takes for your intestines to recover. Any major abdominal surgery on the small or large intestines causes them to "go to sleep." Your surgeon handling the small intestine or colon during the process of removing a segment traumatizes them and causes the intestines to temporarily stop working. This is called *postoperative ileus*. (*Ileus* means "slowing down.") It is a normal response to major abdominal surgery. Postoperative ileus lasts three to five days and is completely reversible. During this period, your intestines will not be able to move liquid waste products toward the anus for removal, so fluid can back up into the stomach. This backup can cause you to feel nauseous and result in vomiting. Food given to you during postoperative ileus will make you feel sick. This is why the nasogastric tube placed down your throat and into your stomach at the time of the operation is left in place. The tube will suck out any fluid that backs up during postoperative ileus.

When your intestines start to become active again, you may hear a lot of growling noises in your abdomen and may

After my diagnosis of colon cancer, my first question was whether I would have to wear a colostomy bag. My surgeon reassured me I would not need one and that the majority of patients do not.

Sally, 57
Survivor

experience gas pains before passing gas. When this occurs, your surgeon may remove the nasogastric tube. Once the tube is removed, you will likely be able to start drinking liquids to see if your stomach can tolerate anything in it. If so, regular food will soon follow. After you start to pass gas, you may experience loose bowel movements that come very suddenly. You may also pass a small amount of blood with initial bowel movements. Both gas and a little bleeding are normal.

Keeping Lungs Expanded

After the operation, the nurses caring for you will tell you to practice deep breathing and coughing. Deep breaths help keep the lungs expanded to prevent pneumonia. If you smoke or have a history of lung disease, deep breathing is especially important. Because deep breathing hurts after major abdominal surgery, it is natural to take short, incomplete breaths. Concentrate on your breathing while recovering in the hospital. An incentive spirometer can assist in expanding your lungs. Keep this device by your bedside and use it often. Placing a pillow on your stomach and holding it as you cough will also ease the pain immediately after surgery.

Blood Tests

For several days after your operation, blood will be taken from your arm each morning to evaluate your blood count and electrolytes. Since these lab values will fluctuate after major abdominal surgery, your surgeon needs to monitor them during recovery.

If your blood count drops too low, you may require a transfusion. A low blood count can lead to low blood pressure, fatigue, and potentially a heart attack if you have a history of heart problems. If electrolytes in the blood drop too low, they can lead to abnormal heart rhythms and seizures and can prolong the inactivity of the intestines following surgery.

Regaining Mobility

Getting out of bed and walking in your room or in the hallway as soon as you are physically able is also important for a fast, uncomplicated recovery. Walking may be difficult while you're connected to various tubes and intravenous lines, but the nurses or a therapist will assist you. Walking gets the blood circulating, prevents blood clots from forming, and may help "wake up" your intestines faster. Walking, like coughing and deep breathing, will cause some initial discomfort. However, as each day passes, it will become easier.

My pain while recovering from surgery was well controlled with the PCA device. I would recommend this to anyone having major abdominal surgery.

Clare, 64
Patient

Planning for Additional Treatment

Before discharge, ask your surgeon about the final pathology report describing the final stage or extent of your colorectal cancer. This report should be available three to four days after your operation. This report will tell your surgeon how far the cancer has spread through the colon wall and whether lymph nodes are involved. If further treatment is needed after surgery, usually your surgeon will call an *oncologist* for consultation. An oncologist is a doctor trained in internal medicine, with specialty training in the medical treatment of cancer. The oncologist is the doctor who gives chemotherapy and treats cancer once the surgeon is finished. Ask your surgeon if you'll need chemotherapy. If you do, an oncologist should come by to discuss your treatment plan prior to discharge.

Discharge from the Hospital

As your hospital stay draws to an end, you should be walking as much as possible and eating normal food. Your bowel movements should be close to normal, and the pain from your incision should be adequately controlled with oral pain medication.

On the day you're discharged from the hospital, you will be given instructions on care of your incision, things to avoid, a prescription for pain medicine, a follow-up appointment with your surgeon and/or oncologist, instructions on bathing and activity level, and any other instructions your surgeon feels you will need. If your surgeon used metal staples to close your incision, they will need to be removed during a follow-up office appointment, usually in seven to ten days. (These staples are different from those used internally to connect the segments of your colon.) Find out when you should return for this and any other follow-up appointments.

Recovering at Home

Recovering at home after colorectal cancer surgery can take four to eight weeks. While at home, it is normal to initially not have much of an appetite. Your appetite will improve over the next several weeks. Feel free to eat what you like. Most people lose ten to twenty pounds following surgery.

Do not expect to have a normal energy level right away. It will take one to two months for your energy to return to the preoperative level. Do not try to do too much too fast. Limit your activities, and do not expect to return to work for at least one month. Expect your energy level to fluctuate, alternating between good days and bad days. This is completely normal after major colorectal surgery.

Your bowel habits should quickly return to normal once you return home despite having part of your colon removed. Persistent diarrhea while at home is *not* normal. Let your surgeon know if this occurs. You must watch out for infection, too. Beware of fever, any drainage, redness, increasing pain from your abdominal incision, and coughing up dark sputum. All these are warning signs of infection, and your surgeon needs to be notified immediately. Persistent nausea, abdominal pain, and vomiting are also not normal and also should be reported.

In addition to being a physical strain, recovering at home from colorectal cancer surgery can be full of mental peaks and valleys. Despite being successfully treated, the fact that you had cancer will be on your mind. You may worry about the cancer coming back. This kind of mental stress is especially prevalent when you are at home, inactive, and recovering with plenty of time to think. Try to keep busy at home with hobbies and things that exercise your mental capabilities. Do not be afraid to open up to family and friends. Talk with them about how you're feeling, your fears and your concerns. Try to maintain a positive outlook. Seek out cancer support groups in your community. They can provide moral support and practical advice for recovery. Talk with friends, neighbors, and coworkers who have had cancer and have been

Recovering from colon surgery definitely has its ups and downs. It took a while to get my normal appetite and energy level back. However, once recovered, I was able to be as active as ever.

Michael, 58
Survivor

successfully treated. Remember, when colorectal cancer is diagnosed and treated early, it is very curable.

Questions to Ask Your Surgeon

- Which operation is best for me?
- How can I prepare for surgery in order to make my recovery complication free?
- What are the possible complications of my operation? What's my risk for complications?
- Did the operation remove all the cancer?
- What is the final stage of my cancer? Will I need further treatment?

7

Radiation Therapy

Radiation therapy is used to treat a variety of cancers in a variety of settings. Radiation kills cancer cells without permanently harming the surrounding normal cells. Cancer cells are chaotic and multiply much faster than normal cells. By dividing faster, cancer cells are more sensitive to the effects of radiation.

Radiation may be used in several ways to treat colorectal cancer. On rare occasions it is the primary treatment, used in place of an operation. Sometimes radiation is used after surgery to kill any cancer cells that were left behind but might not be visible. Often-times radiation is first used to shrink a large, previously unremoveable cancer so a surgeon can remove it more safely. Radiation can also be given in combination with chemotherapy in certain situations. Finally, radiation can be used to treat a cancer if it has spread to other organs, such as the bones.

A *radiation oncologist* usually gives radiation treatments. A radiation oncologist is first trained in internal medicine and then trained in the specialty field of radiation oncology. The treatments are carried out on a daily outpatient basis, usually over five to eight weeks. The treatments take only minutes to deliver.

When Is Radiation Therapy Recommended?

Colon Cancer

For colon cancer, radiation therapy is mainly used after an operation or if the cancer has spread to the bones. If your surgeon feels it is necessary to kill any cells not visible to the naked eye where the cancer was removed, he or she will use radiation therapy. This scenario occurs when, during surgery, a colon cancer is seen growing into neighboring organs like the spleen, bladder, or kidneys. Radiation is indicated if your surgeon feels cancer cells were left behind. In this case, radiation therapy can help prevent the cancer from growing back in the same location.

Radiation therapy is rarely used as a first-line treatment for colon cancer or in place of surgery. It is also not indicated if the lymph nodes are involved with cancer. In this case, chemotherapy, to be discussed in the next chapter, is a better therapy.

Rectal Cancer

Radiation therapy plays a more visible role in the treatment of rectal cancer. As discussed earlier, the rectum is the last six to ten inches of colon leading to the anus. With rectal cancer, radiation therapy can be used either before or after surgery.

As with colon cancer, early diagnosis and surgery offer the best hope for a cure. However, because rectal cancer cells are more susceptible to radiation than colon cancer cells, radiation therapy may be an appropriate treatment. Radiation therapy may be used to shrink a large rectal cancer before an operation. This gives the surgeon a better chance at removing the entire cancer.

Radiation therapy may also be used to shrink a rectal cancer so it can be removed through the anus to avoid a major abdominal operation.

Radiation therapy may also be indicated after surgery of the rectum if your surgeon feels cancer cells not visible to the naked eye may have been left behind. This will help decrease the chance of the cancer returning in the same location. Ask your doctor whether radiation therapy would benefit you.

Types of Radiation Therapy

When you receive radiation treatments, a radiation beam is aimed directly at the part of your body involved with the cancer. Your entire body is not exposed to the radiation beam during the course of the treatments. Focusing the radiation beam at the tumor site kills cancer cells and minimizes the damage to the normal, surrounding cells. A fitted lead body shield provides additional protection to surrounding cells and organs.

For most patients treated for colon cancer, surgery is the main treatment. However, radiation treatment is sometimes used to treat a cancer of the rectum before or after surgery.

Mark, Radiation Oncologist

Before administering the therapy, your radiation oncologist first maps out and marks the direct target site on your body. He or she then fits a lead shield around the site to protect you from the harmful effects of excess radiation.

Radiation therapy is divided into several different types based on how the radiation beam is directed and delivered. Two types, external beam and endocavity radiation, are used to treat colorectal cancers. Your doctor will determine the type of radiation that will work best for you.

External Beam Radiation

External beam radiation is commonly used to treat many different cancers. The beam is directed from outside the body by a large, cone-shaped machine called a *linear accelerator.* The linear accelerator sends the radiation beam directly to the mapped-out area of the body, killing remaining cancer cells. Normal tissues and skin surrounding the targeted area are not in the line of fire.

Normally, external beam radiation is used to treat colon cancer only if the cancer was attached to other organs at the time of its surgical removal and the surgeon feels it was not completely removed. This treatment may also be indicated if, at the time of surgery, it was discovered that the cancer had grown into the abdominal wall. In both instances, external beam radiation reduces the chances of the cancer returning in the same spot.

For rectal cancer, external beam radiation may be used to shrink a large tumor before it is removed with surgery. It may also be used after surgery if your surgeon feels some cancer cells were inadvertently left behind.

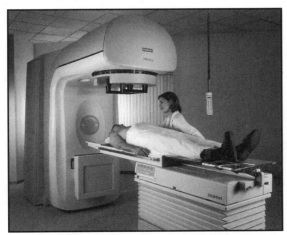

A patient receives an external beam radiation treatment.
Photo courtesy of Sieman's Medical Systems, Inc.

Endocavity Radiation

Another form of external beam radiation, *endocavity radiation,* is primarily used to treat rectal cancer. (It is not used to treat colon cancer.) Here, a linear accelerator focuses a beam of radiation at pinpoint range through the anus at the targeted rectal cancer. The beam can shrink a large tumor prior to surgery and/or kill potential cancer cells left behind after an operation.

Side Effects of Radiation Therapy

The side effects associated with radiation therapy are a result of the radiation beam hitting normal tissues surrounding the targeted area. Any tissue or organ in the path of a radiation beam, including skin, muscle, and any intra-abdominal organ, may be traumatized by radiation. Your radiation oncologist will try to minimize the trauma to normal tissues by tightly focusing the beam and using protective lead shielding. Many of the side effects are treatable, temporary, and go away once the therapy is concluded.

In retrospect, the radiation therapy I received for my cancer was not that bad. The professionals treating me were very patient at explaining the treatment. There were no surprises.

Thelma, 65
Survivor

Skin Irritation

This is one of the most common side effects of radiation therapy. As your radiation therapy progresses, the skin in the beam's path may become dry, irritated, and peel like a sunburn. These changes occur over a period of weeks and may leave your skin permanently rough and darkened. Plan to wear loose clothing during the treatments. Ask your doctor about which creams and lotions to apply.

Fatigue

Many people experience fatigue during radiation therapy. This is due to the overall effect radiation has on the body. It takes time for your body to recover from the trauma of radiation therapy. Expect your energy level to be below normal during treatment. Be sure to get plenty of rest. Also be sure to eat enough calories to keep your energy up. Your fatigue should go away several weeks after you finish therapy.

Nausea and Diarrhea

Nausea and diarrhea are two common side effects of radiation therapy, especially if the radiation is directed at organs inside the abdominal cavity. These side effects can be controlled with medication and should disappear once therapy is over. Make sure to drink plenty of fluids to avoid dehydration.

> *My job is to calm any fears and answer any questions patients may have about their upcoming treatments. I find that an informed patient experiences much less stress.*
>
> *Karen*
> *Nurse*

Rectal Irritation

Rectal irritation is common when the radiation treatments are directed at a cancer of the rectum. The irritation can be treated with creams and should heal once the treatments have stopped.

Bladder Irritation

Like the rectum, the bladder can also be traumatized by radiation treatments. The urinary bladder is close to the rectum. Any radiation directed at a rectal cancer invariably hits the bladder, resulting in infection and/or discomfort with urination. Like most of the side effects of radiation therapy, bladder irritation will go away once therapy is stopped.

Questions to Ask Your Doctor

- Do I need radiation before and/or after my colorectal cancer operation? If so, how will it be given and for how long?

- If I have a cancer of the rectum, can radiation therapy help me avoid a colostomy?

- What are the side effects of my radiation therapy?

- Are these side effects permanent? How can they be treated?

8

Chemotherapy

Chemotherapy—the administration of anticancer drugs—plays a major role in the treatment of all cancers, both before and after surgery. The main goals of chemotherapy are to shrink a cancer, prolong survival, and prevent the cancer from coming back. As mentioned in the last chapter, cancer cells divide much faster than normal cells. Like radiation therapy, chemotherapy primarily targets fast-dividing cancer cells. However, chemotherapy still affects other cells, especially other rapidly dividing normal cells, such as the hair follicles. This is why patients often lose their hair during chemotherapy treatment.

Different cancers are treated with different chemotherapeutic drugs. Your surgeon, in consultation with your other doctors, usually determines if chemotherapy is necessary. If your doctor decides chemotherapy is right for you, he or she will formulate an individualized chemotherapy plan that is designed to treat your specific type of cancer.

Combining Chemotherapy with Other Treatments

In general, chemotherapy can be given in several settings. Where and how your chemotherapy is administered depends on:

- the type of cancer
- whether the cancer can be treated surgically
- the stage of the cancer
- the goals in using chemotherapy
- your overall health

Adjuvant Chemotherapy

Adjuvant chemotherapy is given *after* surgery and in addition to some other treatment. It is used to reduce the risk of the cancer coming back and to improve long-term survival. For colorectal cancer, adjuvant chemotherapy is given if the cancer has spread through the entire wall of the colon. It is also indicated if the lymph nodes are involved with cancer (stage III). As you've learned, when cancer cells spread to the lymph nodes, the cancer cells have the potential to travel through the blood and spread everywhere. Chemotherapy given to patients with lymph node involvement should kill any unseen cancer cells that can potentially spread. Ask your doctor about your stage of colorectal cancer and whether you can benefit from adjuvant chemotherapy.

Chemotherapy is not indicated for everyone. The stage of your cancer, particularly if the lymph nodes are involved, will determine if you need it after surgery.

Marilyn
Oncologist

Neoadjuvant Chemotherapy

Neoadjuvant chemotherapy is given *before* any surgery. Treating some cancers first with chemotherapy and then performing surgery may be beneficial to survival and reduce the chances of the cancer returning. Chemotherapy first can shrink a cancer so it can be completely removed by an operation. Neoadjuvant chemotherapy is not typically used for colon cancer because surgery is such an effective first-line treatment. However, neoadjuvant chemotherapy may be indicated in cancer of the rectum in order to make the surgery more successful.

Palliative Chemotherapy

> *The chemotherapy given to patients today for colorectal cancer is much better tolerated than the drugs given ten years ago.*
> *Kenneth*
> *Oncologist*

When chemotherapy is termed *palliative*, it gives temporary relief from but does not cure a cancer. Chemotherapy may shrink the tumor and slow its growth throughout the body. Palliative chemotherapy may be an option when the cancer has already spread to other organs such as the liver, lungs, or bones at the time of initial diagnosis or at the time of surgery, and is considered incurable. Surgery may or may not play a role depending on the type and location of the cancer.

How Is Chemotherapy Given?

Chemotherapy can be given as a pill or as intravenous (IV) medication. When given by IV, some types of chemotherapy are very hard on the veins in the arm and cause them to break. To avoid this, your surgeon may place a tube called a *Hickman catheter* or *Portacath* inside the large vein in your neck or just underneath your collarbone (*clavicle*). The tube comes out a small incision in your chest and remains in place for as long as it is needed. Chemotherapy is given through the tube, sparing your arm veins. When not in use, the tube is covered with a bandage. Your doctor can place this tube during an outpatient surgical procedure that takes thirty to sixty minutes using local anesthesia with some sedative medicines. When the chemotherapy is finished, your surgeon can remove the catheter in his or her office.

Chemotherapy is usually given to patients with colorectal cancer in an outpatient setting. It rarely requires overnight hospitalization unless complications occur. The chemotherapy is given by a *medical oncologist*, a doctor who specializes in the medical treatment of cancer. This specialist is trained in internal medicine and in oncology. He or she will decide what type of chemotherapy you will receive and how much. During your visits to the oncologist's office, a nurse who specializes in giving chemotherapy connects you to the intravenous chemotherapy while your doctor oversees the procedure.

Side Effects of Chemotherapy

Despite the benefits of chemotherapy for treating colorectal cancer, there are side effects. The type of chemotherapy you receive, the dosage, and the duration of your treatment all impact your side effects. Fortunately, most are temporary and go away once the treatment ends.

The chemotherapy used to treat colorectal cancer is generally well tolerated by most people. Most side effects are mild and can be treated with medication. The following tips for coping with the various side effects are offered by the American Cancer Society.

Diarrhea

This is one of the more common side effects of chemotherapy used to treat colorectal cancer. It is caused by chemotherapy acting on the fast-dividing, normal cells lining the inside of the stomach and intestines. Abdominal cramping can also accompany diarrhea. Both may last several hours to several days and can lead to dehydration.

Drink plenty of fluids. Since diarrhea can cause the body to lose a large amount of water in a short period of time, you can also lose important minerals and electrolytes. Ask your doctor about replacing these. If you're having diarrhea, avoid coffee, tea, alcohol, and sweets. Stay away from high-fiber, greasy, and spicy foods. Eat small amounts of solid food frequently throughout the day. If the diarrhea persists for more than twenty-four hours, call your doctor. Do not take any over-the-counter medicine for diarrhea without consulting your doctor.

When I received my chemotherapy, I thought I would be in the hospital and be sick all the time. To my surprise, I received the treatments as an outpatient and really just felt tired during the experience.
Mary, 56
Survivor

Nausea and Vomiting

Both nausea and vomiting are side effects of chemotherapy used to treat colorectal cancer. The effects of chemotherapy on the cells lining your stomach and certain cells in the brain that control nausea cause these side effects. It is difficult to predict how each person will react to chemotherapy and how long the nausea and vomiting will last.

If you feel nauseous at home, stay hydrated by drinking plenty of water or other liquids. Eat bland food in small amounts and stay away from strong, spicy foods. Ask your doctor about medication that can counteract nausea. If the medication doesn't correct your nausea and vomiting within twenty-four hours, notify your doctor. If the nausea and vomiting persist, you may need to be admitted to the hospital for intravenous fluids and medication. Below are some tips for dealing with nausea or vomiting:

- Eat several small meals during the day to avoid feeling too full.
- Eat and drink slowly. Chew foods well.
- Try eating dry foods like toast or crackers. (Don't try this if you have mouth sores or a dry mouth.)
- Wear loose-fitting clothes.
- Avoid odors that bother you. If the smell of food makes the nausea worse, try staying out of the kitchen while food is being cooked.
- Breathe deeply and slowly when you feel nauseous.
- Suck on ice cubes, mints, or tart candies (unless you have mouth sores).

Hair Loss

Hair loss is another common side effect of chemotherapy. As mentioned earlier, hair loss is caused by damage to the fast-dividing *hair follicles*. Although hair loss can occur anywhere on the body, it is mainly confined to the head. Once the treatments are complete, the hair grows back. However, the hair may grow back in a different color or somewhat different texture. During chemotherapy, some people wear hats, scarves, or wigs to cover their heads and stay warm. If you're experiencing hair loss, protect exposed hairless areas from sun exposure with sunblock and protective clothing.

To cope with hair loss, the American Cancer Society recommends:

- Use mild shampoos.
- Use a soft hair brush.
- Use low heat on your hair dryer.
- Don't use brush rollers to set your hair.
- Don't dye your hair or get a permanent.
- Have your hair cut short. A shorter style will make hair look thicker and fuller.
- Protect your scalp from the sun with a hat, scarf, or sunscreen.

Fatigue

Fatigue is a very common side effect of chemotherapy and can have a number of causes. It can be caused by the chemotherapy's effect on the bone marrow and resulting reduction in red blood cells; this reduction may cause anemia and, in turn, fatigue. Fatigue can also result from dehydration from persistent diarrhea.

Whatever the cause, most patients on chemotherapy experience some degree of fatigue. For some, fatigue occurs around the time of treatments. Others feel fatigued during the entire course of therapy. The fatigue may last even after chemotherapy has ended, and it may take weeks for your body to recover its normal energy. For normally active patients, the fatigue can be a source of frustration, even depression. Try to stay positive and remember that the fatigue is temporary. Here are a few tips for coping with fatigue:

- Limit your activities. Do only those things that are most important to you.

- Take several short naps or breaks during the day.

- Some people find that taking short walks or exercising lightly helps to decrease fatigue.

- Maintain good nutrition. Try to eat a well-balanced diet.

- Ask for help when you need it.

Mouth Sores

Chemotherapy can cause painful sores and ulcers on the lips, mouth, gums, and throat. These sores can become infected. They can also make eating and drinking difficult, which can lead to dehydration. Fortunately, mouth sores disappear once the treatments have concluded. Ask your doctor about medication to treat these sores. Stay hydrated by drinking plenty of water. Avoid spicy, sauce-based foods. Eat soft foods such as baby food, milk shakes, or ice cream until your condition improves. Here are additional suggestions for coping with mouth sores:

I wanted to know what to expect. My doctor was good to explain the side effects of the chemotherapy, and someone from his office was always available when I had questions at home.

Frank, 65
Survivor

- See your dentist if possible before chemotherapy to have your teeth cleaned and any cavities filled.

- Brush and floss your teeth properly, using a soft toothbrush; hard bristles can damage tissues.

- Rinse your toothbrush well after use and store it in a dry place.

- Avoid commercial mouthwashes that contain a lot of salt or alcohol. Ask your doctor or nurse about a mouthwash that you might use. Your dentist may recommend a fluoride rinse or special gel for oral care.

Low Blood Counts

Chemotherapy can damage actively dividing cells in the *bone marrow*. Bone marrow is an important source of red blood cells, infection-fighting white blood cells, and cells that help the blood to clot. By temporarily damaging bone marrow cells, chemotherapy can cause anemia, a low red blood cell count. Chemotherapy can also reduce the number of *platelets*, cells that help clot the blood. If your platelet counts get too low (*thrombocytopenia*), you can bleed or bruise very easily. If you notice unexpected bruises on your body, contact your doctor immediately.

Fortunately, the chemotherapeutic drugs used to treat colorectal cancer have mild effects on bone marrow and do not present a major problem. Once chemotherapy has stopped, the low blood counts are completely treatable and reversible. Your doctor should monitor your blood counts with periodic blood work.

Infections

Chemotherapy can also lower your white blood cell count. This may lead to a weakening of the immune system (*neutropenia*), which makes an individual susceptible to infections. If you're receiving chemotherapy, you are more prone to get infections throughout the body, including pneumonia, blood infections, urine infections, and skin infections. Be alert for the signs of infection—fever over 100 degrees, shaking chills, sweats, coughing up dark or bloody sputum, pain or burning with urination, and pain or redness around cuts. If you feel an infection coming on, notify your doctor immediately. Infections can be effectively treated with antibiotics. To reduce your risk of infection:

- Stay away from people who have diseases that you can catch, such as a cold, the flu, the measles, or chicken pox.
- Wash your hands often during the day, especially after using the bathroom.
- Clean your rectal area gently but thoroughly after each bowel movement. Notify your doctor or nurse if this area becomes irritated or if you have hemorrhoids.
- Stay away from children who have recently received vaccinations.
- Clean cuts and scrapes right away.
- Wear gloves when gardening or cleaning up after pets or small children.
- Use a soft toothbrush that won't hurt your gums.
- Be careful not to cut or nick yourself.

Rashes

Chemotherapy used to treat colorectal cancer can result in rashes on your hands or feet. These rashes can itch and be painful. However, they are temporary. Ask your doctor about medication to relieve the itching. Try to avoid scratching, which can lead to infections requiring antibiotics.

Questions to Ask Your Doctor

- Do I need chemotherapy? If so, how will it help me?

- What will be the duration of chemotherapy? How often will I be treated?
- Will chemotherapy help me live longer and prevent the cancer from returning?
- What specific side effects need I be aware of?
- What can I do to minimize these side effects and when should I notify you?

9

Clinical Trials

You've probably heard media reports about new cancer treatments. You probably have a number of questions about them: Where do these new treatments come from? How do doctors know if they work? How do people qualify for these treatments? New cancer treatments often take many years to become available to most patients. Before approval, they must undergo *clinical trials*, studies that test their effectiveness in people. The goal of a clinical trial, particularly in the treatment of cancer, is to compare a new, potentially better treatment to one that is currently the standard of care. Today, there are hundreds of ongoing clinical trials involving thousands of patients in an attempt to cure a variety of diseases. Many of these trials are focused on finding new ways to treat cancer with new and improved drugs.

U.S. clinical trials are carried out under the auspices and regulations of the Food and Drug Administration (FDA). Most clinical trials are carried out by doctors based at large university hospitals in major cities across the country. Patients who participate in clinical trials volunteer to test new drugs and/or procedures that have already undergone extensive laboratory evaluation and appear more potent than standard therapy. Clinical trials are divided into three phases, each designed to give doctors different types of information.

A *phase I* clinical trial helps doctors determine the safest dose of a new drug/procedure, one that will produce the greatest benefit with the fewest side effects. This study exposes people to the new treatment for the first time.

Phase II clinical trial determines if the new drug/procedure actually shrinks cancer in patients. It also helps determine how many patients receive a positive response from the new treatment.

If the new treatment has acceptable side effects (determined in phase I) and shrinks tumors (determined in phase II), then it moves on to *phase III*. A phase III clinical trial compares the new treatment to existing treatments. If the new drug/procedure is found to be more effective in treating cancer than the standard therapy, it will go in front of the FDA for clinical approval. Once the FDA approves the treatment, it becomes available to doctors to prescribe to their patients.

Are You a Candidate for a Clinical Trial?

The best way to find out if you can be part of a cancer clinical trial is to ask your surgeon or oncologist. Patients must meet criteria that have been established for each clinical trial. Your doctor can find out what the criteria are and help you determine whether you qualify. For cancer trials, most patients must have advanced cancer at the time of diagnosis that has not responded to standard treatment or have a recurrence of cancer. Most have already undergone surgery and have been treated with conventional chemotherapy and/or radiation.

If conventional therapy is not working for you, then you may be a candidate for a clinical trial. Ask your doctor about the latest studies and advances in chemotherapy. You can also get a list of current clinical trials by calling the National Cancer Institute's Cancer Information Service at 1-800-4-CANCER. Also, see the Resources section in the back of this book.

Colorectal Cancer and Clinical Trials

For most patients with colorectal cancer, clinical trials aren't an issue. That's because surgery is very effective in treating and potentially curing most patients. Surgery offers a 90 percent or better cure rate when colorectal cancer is diagnosed early. When a colorectal cancer has spread to neighboring lymph nodes, chemotherapy is very effective in prolonging survival. Even if a cancer returns several years after treatment, chemotherapy is often effective in shrinking it and prolonging survival. However, if your colorectal cancer is not responding to surgery and/or conventional therapy, participating in a clinical trial may be a treatment option for you.

Future Chemotherapy: New Hope on the Horizon

Several new and exciting drug treatments for colorectal cancer are currently being investigated in clinical trials. Many of these new drugs are very specific, attacking only cancer cells, not normal cells. By targeting only cancer cells, many of the side effects that are currently a problem with chemotherapy could be eliminated.

Angiogenesis inhibitors are drugs that choke off the blood supply to cancer cells. These drugs do not affect normal cells. By blocking the blood supply, the nutrient supply is cut off, killing the cancerous cells.

Very specific proteins called *monoclonal antibodies* seek out and destroy cancer cells. Monoclonal antibodies are normally produced in the body in response to a foreign invader, such as a virus or bacteria. Researchers can now produce specific antibodies in the lab that target only colon cancer cells as foreign invaders. These antibodies act as assassins, killing only their cancer cell targets and leaving normal cells alone.

Cancer vaccines stimulate the body's immune system. These vaccines act much like the ones we received as children. However, instead of preventing deadly infections like polio, cancer vaccines prevent the spread or recurrence of colorectal cancer.

Questions to Ask Your Doctor

- Am I a candidate for a clinical trial?
- What is the purpose of the study?
- What kinds of tests and treatments does the study involve?
- What does the treatment do?
- What are my choices if I decide not to participate in the clinical trial?
- Will I have to be hospitalized for the study?
- What are the risks and potential benefits of participating in this study?
- What type of long-term follow-up care is part of the study?

10

Follow-Up Care

Once you are diagnosed with colorectal cancer, or any cancer for that matter, there is a chance that the cancer may recur. Consequently, it is important that you be alert for any changes in your body that may indicate the recurrence of cancer so your doctor can diagnose and treat it early.

A recurrence can occur at a different location in your colon, at a site near where part of your colon was removed, or in the liver, lungs, spine, lining of the abdominal cavity, ovaries, adrenal glands, or brain. The liver is the most common organ where a colorectal cancer can recur years after your initial operation. Approximately 50,000 patients are diagnosed with a liver recurrence each year.

Your risk of recurrence is directly related to the stage of your cancer at the time of initial diagnosis. A cancer caught early and confined to the colorectal wall is less likely to recur than a cancer involving the lymph nodes at the time of initial diagnosis.

Symptoms of Colorectal Cancer Recurrence

- *Change in Bowel Habits:* Prolonged constipation not responsive to laxatives, abdominal pain, persistent diarrhea, or a change in stool caliber.

- *Rectal Bleeding:* Passing dark or bright red blood with bowel movements, or a change in stool color.

- *Persistent Urge to Have a Bowel Movement:* Urge to have a bowel movement despite just having had a bowel movement (tenesmus).

- *Excess Mucus Secretion:* With bowel movements.

- *Chronic Abdominal Pain, Bloating, and Fullness*

- *Decreased Appetite, Fatigue, and Weight Loss:* May be indicative of a recurrence in the liver or other organs.

- *Jaundice:* A yellowing of the eyes or skin may be indicative of a recurrence in the liver.

- *New Joint or Bone Pain:* Onset of acute back or rib pain may be indicative of a recurrence in the spine.

Detecting Cancer Recurrence

After initial treatment, your doctor will devise a follow-up plan for the next two years. This plan will consist of periodic checkups, blood tests, X-rays, and other procedures, such as a colonoscopy. All these tests are designed to detect a recurrence at its earliest stage. After two years, your plan will be changed to reflect your decreased risk of recurrence. It will be changed again at five and ten years after treatment. During your first follow-up visit with your doctor, ask him or her about your follow-up detection plan.

Periodic Checkups

Once you've been treated for colorectal cancer, your doctor will follow your health closely for the rest of your life. During the first two years after treatment, you should see your doctor every three months. During these checkups, he or she will perform a physical examination and check for blood in your stool, looking for evidence of recurrence. After two years, the checkups will be spaced further apart since your recurrence risk decreases over time.

Blood Tests

During your doctor visits, your blood will be drawn periodically for testing. Blood tests are usually performed every six months for the first two years of follow-up and then once a year. Blood tests help monitor your red blood cell count since a low count (anemia) is a sign of recurrence. Since the liver is a common site of recurrence, it will also be evaluated periodically with the same blood tests that were performed before your surgery. Your doctor will also perform a blood test every three to four months to measure your carcinoembryonic antigen (CEA) level. As mentioned previously, CEA is a protein produced by some cancers, including colorectal cancer. Elevated blood levels of CEA may be an indication that the cancer has come back. If your doctor finds a high CEA level, he or she will perform other tests to investigate further. A table of blood tests and their corresponding measurements appear in the appendix in the back of this book.

X-rays and Scans

If your doctor suspects your colorectal cancer has returned, he or she will try to confirm this with X-ray tests. A CT scan is usually carried out to look for recurrence in the liver, lungs, or abdominal cavity. (An MRI is a similar test and provides similar information regarding recurrence in internal organs.) If a CT scan is done and a cancer nodule is identified in your liver, a radiologist may perform a CT-guided needle biopsy of it for diagnosis. An ultrasound may also be used to evaluate your liver for the possibility of cancer recurrence. A chest X-ray may also be done to evaluate the possible recurrence of the cancer in the lungs. A bone scan is used to evaluate the possibility of a recurrence in the bones.

Once you are told you have cancer, your entire outlook on life changes. Thankfully, I was successfully treated and now enjoy the everyday things I used to take for granted.
Julie, 63
Survivor

A PET scan (positron emission tomography) may also be used to see if a cancer is present in other organs in the abdominal cavity. This scan relies on cancer cells ability to absorb glucose more rapidly than normal cells. Prior to the scan, the patient drinks a radioactive glucose-like solution. Then, if cancer cells are present, they will show up in the scan, having absorbed the glucose solution.

Colonoscopy

In addition to periodic office examinations, blood tests, and X-rays, you will also need a colonoscopy every year after your initial treatment. Colonoscopy is necessary to detect polyps or cancer recurrence early on.

What If the Cancer Returns?

If your colorectal cancer does return, there are several treatment options. These options include another operation, chemotherapy, radiation therapy, cryoablation, radio-frequency ablation, and portal vein infusion. The options that are right for you will depend on where the cancer is located.

Surgery

If your surgeon determines you are a candidate for surgery, another operation may be the best curative measure. Surgery has the best chance of being successful if the recurrent tumor is isolated to one organ and confined to one area of that organ. If, for instance, you have a solitary tumor that is confined to one part of your liver, then surgery to remove a portion of your liver is the best option since it has shown to improve survival over chemotherapy. If the cancer comes back in a different part of your colon, then surgery again is the best option. Or, if you have a single tumor that is confined to a single area of your lung, surgery is also the best option.

If colorectal cancer has come back in several areas of one organ, such as the liver, then surgery is not the best treatment. In this case, other treatments such as cryoablation or radio-frequency ablation are possible options. *Cryoablation* involves the placement of a probe, either surgically or under the guidance of a CT scan, into the middle of the tumor and first freezing it with liquid nitrogen. Once the tumor is frozen, heat is immediately applied to thaw it. The combination of freezing and thawing is effective for killing tumor cells without harming normal surrounding cells. *Radio-frequency ablation* is a similar procedure. It involves the placement of a probe in the middle of the tumor and killing the cancer cells with thermal energy.

If your cancer recurrence involves multiple organs, then chemotherapy in combination with radiation therapy may be the best option. Chemotherapy can be directly given to the liver, sparing the rest of the body of side effects. This direct infusion of chemotherapy is given through a catheter surgically inserted in the main blood vessel entering the liver. The technique is called *portal vein infusion*. Chemotherapy may also be used after surgical removal of your recurrent cancer to kill any unseen cells that may have been left behind.

Radiation therapy is commonly used when colorectal cancer comes back in the bones. It may also be used when a cancer of the rectum recurs close to where it was initially removed.

Living with a Colostomy

In the beginning, having a colostomy was a major adjustment emotionally and physically. However, I was thankful my rectal cancer was caught early and now I am determined to get back to a normal life.
Sophie, 61
Survivor

More than 750,000 people in the United States with colostomies live normal, active lives and are potentially cured of their cancer. Having an external fecal bag does not mean your lifestyle needs to change dramatically. Initially, a colostomy presents physical and emotional challenges. However, with the proper education and support, these challenges can be overcome. Once recovered from your operation, you can exercise, wear normal clothes, and return to work.

How the Colostomy Is Fitted

If you have a colostomy, many times its location on your abdomen will be determined before surgery by an *enterostomal nurse*. Most hospitals have one or more enterostomal nurses on staff. The nurse will explain how to care for your colostomy, where to get supplies, and how to contact local support groups. You'll find the information and support he or she can provide while you are in the hospital recovering very helpful.

In most patients, the colostomy is located below and to the left of the navel. Health-care professionals refer to this as the left, lower quadrant of the abdomen. It is rare to find colostomies located elsewhere on the abdomen.

To attach the pouch, an individual first places a plastic adhesive barrier (shaped like a doughnut) around the stoma, the opening in the abdomen. This barrier sticks to the skin and protects it from the fecal material leaving the colostomy. This barrier remains in place indefinitely and is changed as it wears down. The external plastic pouch that collects the fecal material is then attached to the adhesive barrier by snapping it in place. The pouch hangs down under your clothes and is usually not noticeable to others.

Colostomy Care

Caring for your colostomy at home is not difficult. The pouch needs to be emptied into the toilet periodically during the day as it fills up. You can empty the pouch by opening a plastic clip at its base and allowing the fecal material to spill into the toilet. Once emptied, the plastic clip can be reattached and the bottom of the pouch closed. Most patients become very adept at emptying the pouch and do not have problems with soiled garments or lingering odors. Patients can insert drops of deodorizer into the bag immediately after it is emptied each time. There are several liquid deodorizers on the market that may be purchased at any medical supply store.

You can exert some control over your colostomy bowel habits by modifying your diet. By watching what you eat and eating at regular intervals, you can control when your colostomy works during the day. You do *not* need to be on a special diet with a colostomy. However, certain foods can affect the consistency of your colostomy output. Some foods may cause diarrhea and/or excess gas. Other foods may cause constipation. Ask your doctor for a referral to a dietician to better understand how foods affect your colostomy.

Periodic checkups and testing is crucial to detecting a cancer recurrence early. Write down a follow-up plan with your doctor and stick to it.

Tess
Nurse

Irrigating your colostomy with a simple saline solution will be helpful if it becomes clogged. Esssentially, colostomy irrigation works like an enema. Ask your nurse or doctor about irrigation and how to do it. The plastic pouch itself usually needs to be replaced every five to seven days. The colostomy opening may be washed with soap and water.

Most persons with colostomies keep extra supplies nearby, such as in the car, just in case they are needed unexpectedly. Make sure you have a generous supply at home. Colostomy supplies can be obtained in some drug stores and in many medical supply stores.

Emotional Support

At first, accepting the fact that you have a colostomy may be emotionally difficult. You may experience feelings of depression, frustration, anger, sadness, and isolation. You may withdraw from family and friends. It's important to realize that all these feelings and reactions are perfectly natural and very common. Talk with your family and friends about your feelings. Let your doctor know how your colostomy is making you feel. Consider seeking out cancer and colostomy support groups in your area. They can provide valuable insights and help you cope with your new situation. For the names and addresses of support groups, see Resources in the back of this book.

Most patients, once they accept having a colostomy, are more readily able to incorporate change into their lives. It will help to concentrate on the positive things. Remember, your cancer is gone and, because of your colostomy, you can now resume living a full life.

Colostomy's Effect on Sexual Activity

Many people wonder if a colostomy will affect their sex lives. Women normally have no loss of sexual function due to colostomy. However, some men who've had colostomies experience a loss of semen during ejaculation. It is possible that a man will have no emission during ejaculation, or he may have a *retrograde emission*, in which the semen is forced backward into the bladder. Why does this occur? Tiny nerves located deep in the pelvis, near the rectum, may be damaged during surgery. Surgeons try to avoid damaging these nerves, but if damage occurs, the emission of semen may be affected. A man's ability to attain an erection is not changed, but pleasurable sensations during sexual activity may be slightly diminished. Still, with a few changes, most individuals adapt and continue having a normal sex life.

Questions to Ask Your Doctor

- How often will I need follow-up care over the next two years?

- What are the chances of my cancer coming back in the next two years?

- What was my latest CEA level? Is it stable or rising?

- Will I need a colonoscopy every year for the rest of my life?

- Are there any new tests on the horizon to detect cancer recurrence early?

11

Prevention and Early Detection

If you are willing to take an active role in your health, medical studies show that you can actually prevent colorectal cancer. In fact, if everyone adhered to the specific diet and lifestyle guidelines and screening recommendations of the American Cancer Society, the incidence of colorectal cancer would be dramatically reduced. In addition, those with the disease would be diagnosed early and have a good chance of being cured with treatment.

Remember that screening is essential for early detection. The earlier colorectal cancer is diagnosed, the better the chance for cure. Studies repeatedly show that annual screening for colorectal cancer prolongs survival and saves lives. In addition, annual screening actually reduces your risk of getting colorectal cancer by up to 20 percent. It does this by detecting precancerous polyps and removing them before they turn cancerous. Unfortunately, today only about a third of people who should undergo screening actually do. This is why colorectal cancer remains the second largest cancer killer.

SCREENING GUIDELINES FOR COLORECTAL POLYPS AND CANCER

Risk	Procedure	Age to Begin	Interval
Average			
• age 50 years or older • no other risk factors	FOBT plus flexible sigmoidoscopy or total colon examination	30	FOBT plus flexible sigmoidoscopy every 3 years DCBE every 5-10 years colonoscopy every 10 years
Moderate			
• prior adenomatous polyps • prior cancer	colonoscopy or	at time of diagnosis	every 3 years
• family history under age 60 years	DCBE	within one year after surgery	every 3 years
		age 40	every 5 years
High			
• familial polyposis	endoscopy	puberty	every 1-2 years
• HNPCC	colonoscopy	age 21	every 1-3 years
• IBD	colonoscopy	about 10 years after diagnosis	every 1-3 years

FOBT: Fecal Occult Blood Testing
DCBE: Double Contrast Barium Enema
HNPCC: Hereditary Non-polyposis Colon Cancer
Reprinted by permission of the American Cancer Society

How Do I Prevent Colorectal Cancer?

- Recognize your personal risk, family history, and get screened.
- Eat a diet high in fruits and vegetables, low in red meat, and high in fiber.

- Take a multivitamin to ensure enough calcium and selenium in your diet.

- Get daily exercise.

- Stop smoking.

- Postmenopausal women should ask their doctors about the benefits of hormone supplements.

- Ask your doctor about taking an aspirin a day for your heart and colon.

Screening Procedures

Annual Checkup

According to the American Cancer Society, the average 50-year-old with no symptoms and no risk factors should undergo yearly screening for colorectal cancer. Such screening starts with a yearly digital rectal examination and testing for fecal occult blood.

If the cancer is caught early, greater than 90% of patients can be cured and live active, normal lives into ripe old age.

*Joseph
Surgeon*

Flexible Sigmoidoscopy and Colonoscopy

In addition, a flexible sigmoidoscopy should be performed every three to five years and a colonoscopy every ten years. If the test for fecal occult blood is positive or a flexible sigmoidoscopy finds polyps in the sigmoid colon or rectum, a full colonoscopy is necessary to examine the rest of the colon. If the colonoscopy finds a polyp and it is successfully removed, it should be repeated in three years since polyps can grow back. Studies have shown that if a precancerous polyp is found in your sigmoid colon or rectum during a routine screening flexible sigmoidoscopy, there is a 6 to 7 percent chance of finding an actual cancer in the part of your colon not reached by the sigmoidoscope. These same studies have also shown that if your screening flexible sigmoidoscopy is totally normal and no polyps are found, you still have a 1.5 to 3 percent chance of having an unsuspected cancer somewhere else in your colon. As a result, doctors are now considering colonoscopy a better screening test than flexible sigmoidoscopy.

Further proof supporting the use of colonoscopy over flexible sigmoidoscopy comes from the National Polyp Study. This study had doctors performing a screening colonoscopy in the average-risk person every three years and removing polyps when found. Over a six-year period in 1,400 patients, 20 to 48 colorectal cancers should have been found given the incidence of the disease in the general population. However, only five cancers were found in the entire patient group. Why so few? The thinking is, since most colorectal cancers come from polyps, by periodically screening for and removing polyps by colonoscopy before they turn cancerous, you can dramatically reduce the incidence of the disease.

Guidelines for Patients at Greater Risk

For patients with a moderate risk factor as defined by the American Cancer Society, such as a family member with a history of colorectal cancer before age 60, screening should start at age 40. This screening should start with a full colonoscopy and continue every three years for life.

For patients with high risk factors as defined by the American Cancer Society, such as an inherited disease that predisposes you to the formation of thousands of precancerous polyps (familial polyposis), a screening colonoscopy should start at puberty and continue every one to two years for life.

Genetic Testing

An estimated 10 percent of all colorectal cancers involve inherited genes. If you have a strong family history of colorectal cancer, such as several members diagnosed before age 60, genetic tests are now available that can predict your risk of developing the disease later in life. These genetic tests involve sampling your blood and analyzing your DNA. A simple blood test can identify abnormal gene mutations. If you test positive for these genetic mutations, you have an 80 percent higher risk than the average person of developing colorectal cancer as you get older. If are at risk, ask your doctor about these tests. By knowing your risk, you and your doctor can develop an aggressive screening program that can detect cancer early or prevent it altogether.

New Tests in Development

Researchers are also developing a new screening test that examines cells shed in the stool of patients. By analyzing the DNA of these cells, doctors can identify genetic changes characteristic of precancerous polyps and colon cancer at their earliest stages. Stool DNA testing will be simple, noninvasive, and accurate. Ask your doctor about this and other new technologies that may become available for screening and preventing colorectal cancer.

Lifestyle Guidelines to Prevent Colon Cancer

Diet

Diet plays a major role in the development of many cancers, including colorectal cancer. It is well known that colorectal cancer is primarily a disease of Western industrialized countries like the United States and Canada. The lifetime risk of getting the disease in Western countries is 6 percent. The incidence of the disease in countries like Japan is much lower. This is thought to be due to differences in diet and exposure to carcinogens. According to some studies, by adhering to a healthful diet, you can reduce your risk of colorectal cancer by up to 50 percent.

Reducing your intake of red meat, cholesterol, and saturated fatty acids can go a long way in preventing precancerous polyps and colorectal cancer. A diet high in fruits and vegetables (five one-half cup servings daily) can also help prevent the formation of polyps and cancer. Fruits and vegetables—particularly the green, leafy type—contain antioxidants, compounds that protect cells against cancer-causing agents in our diet and in the environment. Antioxidants include vitamins A, C, and E. Carotenoids, lycopene, and lutein are other antioxidants commonly found in fruits and vegetables.

My whole life has changed since my colon cancer surgery. I now eat right, stopped smoking, and even exercise daily. I feel good and will do anything to keep the cancer from coming back.

Steven, 55
Survivor

Fiber

It is believed that a diet high in fiber protects against a variety of benign diseases of the colon, such as diverticulosis, in addition to helping lower blood cholesterol levels. The traditional thinking is, fiber also helps prevent colorectal cancer. Fiber dilutes carcinogens in our diet that ultimately make their way to the colon. Fiber also decreases the time the inner lining of the colon is exposed to carcinogens. By minimizing the exposure of the inner lining to potential cancer-causing agents, fiber can prevent DNA mutations that ultimately lead to colorectal cancer.

Calcium

Some studies have suggested a diet deficient in calcium increases your risk of developing polyps and colorectal cancer. One study showed a 20 percent reduction in the incidence of colorectal cancer in patients taking calcium supplements. Calcium appears to block the effects of some carcinogens found in our colon and prevent polyp and cancer formation. If you are not getting enough calcium in your diet, ask your doctor about taking supplements. This is especially important for women, particularly postmenopausal women. Many postmenopausal women take calcium supplements for osteoporosis, or bone loss, as they get older.

Selenium

Selenium is an antioxidant found in the soil and ingested in our diet. It is now becoming clear that a diet deficient in selenium is associated with an increased risk of several cancers, including prostate and colorectal cancer. One study showed a marked decrease in the incidence of colorectal cancer in patients taking daily selenium supplements. Ask your doctor about the benefits of selenium supplements.

Exercise

Studies have shown that a lack of physical activity increases the risk of getting colorectal cancer. Studies also confirm the benefits of daily vigorous exercise in preventing colorectal cancer. Daily exercise is helpful in preventing many other diseases as well, such as heart and lung disease. Try to get at least thirty minutes of exercise, such as brisk walking, every day.

Smoking

Smoking, we know, causes lung cancer. Smoking also contributes to many other cancers, including colorectal cancer. As technology to analyze the DNA in genes becomes more advanced, the link between smoking and colorectal cancer becomes stronger. Medical data suggests smoking can have a damaging effect on the DNA of colon cells, predisposing them to becoming cancerous. By smoking, your risk for a number of noncancerous diseases also increases. If you smoke, talk with your doctor about strategies to quit, including the use of prescription drugs and nicotine patches.

Hormone Therapy

There is emerging evidence that women who take hormone supplements, estrogen and progesterone, have a reduced risk of getting colorectal cancer. This evidence comes mainly from the millions of postmenopausal women who take hormone supplements to reduce the risk of osteoporosis—weakening of the bones—and heart disease. More research will be needed to confirm this benefit.

Aspirin and Other Medications

Aspirin and similar medications can prevent the formation of polyps and colorectal cancer. Over the last three decades, several large studies have focused on people taking an aspirin a day to reduce the risk of heart disease. Surprisingly, these studies show that individuals who take a daily aspirin also have a 40 to 50 percent reduction in the risk of polyps and colorectal cancer. Researchers believe aspirin somehow reverses the precancerous changes in growing precancerous polyps.

Other aspirin-like medications, including ibuprofen, have the same effect. Ibuprofen is a *nonsteroidal anti-inflammatory agent*, or *NSAID*. They are primarily used to treat the pain and inflammation associated with arthritis. They work in normal cells by blocking two enzymes, *Cox-1 and Cox-2*. The Cox-2 enzyme is involved in the transformation of a benign polyp into a precancerous polyp and eventually into a cancer. Today, there are several new arthritis medications on the market that block only the Cox-2 enzyme. There are several ongoing clinical trials looking at the benefits of these new drugs and aspirin in preventing colorectal polyps and cancer. Ask your doctor about them and whether you should be taking an aspirin a day.

Questions to Ask Your Doctor

- What can I do to minimize my risk of getting colorectal cancer?
- What foods should I avoid and what foods can help prevent colorectal cancer?
- How can I stop smoking?
- What is the best exercise program for me to reduce my risk for colorectal cancer?
- Should I be taking an aspirin a day?
- What is the latest research on new drugs that may prevent polyps and colorectal cancer?

Appendix

TNM Staging System for Colorectal Cancer

The following table provides a more thorough listing of TNM stages. The International Staging System describes the extent of spread of a malignant tumor according to the tumor-lymph node-metastasis (TNM) descriptions.

T Tumor

> T1 corresponds to tumor invading mucosa and submucosa.
> T2 corresponds to tumor invading muscularis layer.
> T3 corresponds to tumor invading through muscularis into serosa.
> T4 corresponds to tumor invading through serosa into adjacent organs.

N Nodes

> N0 designates no nodal involvement with cancer.
> N1 designates cancer involving 1 to 3 lymph nodes.
> N2 designates cancer involving 4 or more lymph nodes.

M Metastatic disease

> M0 designates no evidence of metastatic disease.
> M1 designates evidence of spread to distant organs.

Stage	TNM Classification	5-Year Survival Rate
I	T1N0M0	
	T2N0M0	85-95 percent
II	T3N0M0	
	T4N0M0	60-80 percent
III	Any T, N1M0	
	Any T, N2M0	30-60 percent
IV	Any T, Any N, M1	less than 5 percent

Other Staging Systems

Dukes System

The Dukes system uses letters to describe the extent of tumor growth through the colon wall.

Dukes A: Tumor is confined to the colorectal wall. Corresponds to stage I of the TNM system.

Dukes B: Tumor has spread to the lymph nodes surrounding the colorectal wall. Corresponds to Stages II and III of the TNM system.

Dukes C: Tumor has spread to other organs in the body. Corresponds to stage IV of the TNM system.

Kirklin System

A modification of the Dukes system, the Kirklin system uses numbered letters to describe the specific extent of tumor growth through the colorectal wall.

Kirklin A: Tumor growing into but not through the submucosal layer. No lymph nodes involved.

Kirklin B1:   Tumor growing into the muscularis layer but not through it. No lymph nodes involved.

Kirklin B2:   Tumor growing through all layers of the colorectal wall. No lymph nodes involved.

Kirklin C1:   Tumor involving all layers of the colorectal wall except the outermost layer (serosa). However, adjacent lymph nodes are involved.

Kirklin C2:   Tumor growing through all layers, including the serosa, and involving adjacent lymph nodes.

Kirklin D: Tumor metastasized, or spread, to distant organs in the body.

Lab Tests to Detect Colorectal Cancer

The following blood tests are commonly ordered by doctors to check for the presence of colorectal cancer. These tests can also help determine whether a cancer has spread to the liver or other parts of the body. These same tests may also be used to check for any recurrence of cancer. Ask your doctor what the numbers mean. Compare the normal values listed here to your test results.

Complete Blood Count (CBC)	Normal Range
White Blood Cell Count (WBC)	4.0-11 1000/ul
Hemoglobin (Hg)	13-17 g/dl
Hematocrit (Hct)	40-51 percent
Platelets (Plt)	140-200 1000/ul

Electrolytes

Sodium (Na)	141-150 mmol/l
Potassium (K)	3.5-5.2 mmol/l
Chloride (Cl)	98-110 mmol/l
Carbon Dioxide (CO)	24-32 mmol/l

Liver Enzyme Tests

Bilirubin (Bili)	0.2-1.4 mg/dl
Alkaline Phosphatase (Alk Phos)	30-122 u/l
SGOT (AST)	0-41 u/l
SGPT (ALT)	0-41 u/l
Albumin (Alb)	3.5-5.0 g/dl
Lactic Dehydrogenase (LDH)	60-245 u/l
Carcinoembryonic Antigen (CEA)	0.0-3.0 ng/ul

Chemotherapy Drugs for Colorectal Cancer

Fluorouracil (5-FU)

This is the main drug used to treat colorectal cancer involving the lymph nodes and other organs. It is given intravenously. Its side effects include fatigue, nausea, vomiting, hair loss, neutropenia, thrombocytopenia, mucositis, infections, joint pain, depression, and decreased appetite.

Leucovorin

This chemotherapeutic agent is also commonly used to treat colorectal cancer. It is given in combination with fluorouracil because both work better together. The drug is given either by mouth or intravenously. Its side effects include a rash and allergic reaction.

Irinotecan (CPT-11, Camptosar)

This is a new drug to treat colorectal cancer. It is given alone or in combination with fluorouracil or leucovorin. It is given intravenously and has the following side effects: diarrhea, nausea, vomiting, mucositis, neutropenia, and infections.

Oxaliplatin

A relatively new chemotherapeutic drug, oxaliplatin is given in combination with fluorouracil and leucovorin. It is given intravenously and has the following side effects: neutropenia, thrombocytopenia, fatigue, nausea, hair loss, and numbness/tingling in the hands and feet exacerbated by cold temperatures.

5-Fluorouracil Analogues

These drugs are similar to 5-fluorouracil and are considered the next generation of new drugs. They include *Tomudex, Capecitabine (Xeloda), UFT,* and *Ethynyluracil.* Their side effects are similar to 5-fluorouracil and their killing effects on cancer cells may be better.

Monoclonal Antibodies

This class of experimental drugs to treat colorectal cancer are very specific and have minimal side effects on normal cells. They are being tested for their effectiveness on advanced colorectal cancer cells by stopping their growth and blocking their blood supply. The monoclonal antibodies currently being tested include *17-1A, anti-VEGF, and C225.*

Other Drugs

Vaccines

Vaccines are currently being tested in clinical trials to stimulate the body's own immune system to attack and kill colorectal cancer in patients with advanced disease.

Cox-2 Inhibitors

As mentioned in the text, drugs on the market to treat arthritic pain are now being tested to prevent the formation of precancerous polyps and colorectal cancer. These drugs act by blocking an enzyme, Cox-2, vital to the formation of cancer cells and include *aspirin, celebrex, and vioxx.*

Resources

American Cancer Society
15999 Clifton Rd NE
Atlanta, GA 30329-4251
Phone: 1-800-ACS-2345 (1-800-227-2345)
www.cancer.org
With more than two million volunteers and 3,400 local units, this organization works to eliminate cancer as a major health problem through prevention, saving lives and diminishing suffering through research, education, patient services, advocacy, and rehabilitation.

Cancer Care, Inc.
275 7th Ave.
New York, NY 10001
Phone: 212-302-2400 (1-800-813-HOPE)
www.cancercare.org
A nonprofit organization since 1944, Cancer Care offers emotional support, information and practical help to people with all types of cancer and their loved ones. All services are free. Forty-five oncology social workers are available for phone consultations in which they provide emotional counseling and support; Cancer Care also offers education seminars, teleconferences, and referrals to other services.

Wound Ostomy, Continence Nurses Society (WOCN)

1550 S. Coast Highway Suite 201
Laguna Beach, CA 92651
Ph. 888-224-9626
www.wocn.org
This association of nurses provides acute and rehabilitative care for
people with disorders of gastrointestinal, genitourinary, and
integumentary systems. The enterostomal (ET) nurse provides
direct patient care to persons with abdominal stomas, fistulas,
drains, pressure sores, and incontinence. As an educator,
consultant, researcher, and administrator, the ET nurse plays a
pivotal role in the guidance of optimum patient care.

United Ostomy Association (UOA)

19772 MacArthur Blvd. Suite 200
Irvine, CA 92612
1-800-826-0826
www.uoa.org
The United Ostomy Association (UOA) was formed in 1962 to help
ostomy patients return to normal living through mutual aid and
moral support, education in proper ostomy care and management,
exchange of ideas, assistance in improving ostomy equipment and
supplies, advancement of knowledge of gastrointestinal diseases,
cooperation with other organizations having common purposes,
exhibits at medical and public meetings, and public education
about ostomy. Trained members often visit ostomy patients in
hospitals and in their homes to offer moral support and assistance.
Monthly meetings provide information on adjusting to living with
an ostomy.

National Cancer Institute
National Institutes of Health
Bethesda, MD 20892
301-496-4000
1-800-4-CANCER (1-800-422-6237)
www.nci.nih.gov
National institution providing the most recent advances in cancer diagnosis and treatment. Ask for the *Physicians Data Query* to access information on cancer specialists.

American College of Surgeons
633 North St. Clair Street
Chicago, IL 60611
312-302-5000

American Society of Colon and Rectal Surgeons
85 W. Algonquin Road
Suite 550
Arlington Heights, IL 60005
800-791-0001

American College of Gastroenterology
4900-B South 31st Street
Arlington, VA 22206
703-820-7400

American Gastroenterological Association
7910 Woodmont Avenue
7th Floor
Bethesda, MD 20814
301-654-2055

National Hospice Organization (NHO)
1901 North Moore Street, Suite 901
Arlington VA 22209
(703) 243-5900
www.nch.org

Hospice Association of America
National Association of Home Care (NAHC)
228 Seventh Street, SE
Washington, DC 20003-4360
(202) 546-4759
www.hospice-america.org

Association of Oncology Social Work
47000 Westlake Avenue
Glenview, IL 60025-1485
(847) 375-4721
www.aosw.org
Provides information on social workers who are involved in the care of cancer patients.

American Academy of Hospice and Palliative Medicine
P.O. Box 14288
Gainesville, FL 32604-2288
(352) 377-8900
www.aahpm.org

Hospice Nurses Association
Medical Center East, Suite 375
211NorthWhitfield Street
Pittsburgh, PA 15206-3031
(412) 361-2470
www.hpna.org

MEDLINEplus
http://www.nlm.nih.gov/medlineplus
Designed for the public, this site offers an up-to-date collection of consumer health-care information from the world's largest medical library, the U.S. National Library of Medicine at the National Institutes of Health. It is free to consumers, health-care professionals, and scientists. MEDLINEplus web site also lists dozens of links to health organizations.

American Association of Cancer Research
This site provides access to cancer-oriented literature and medical articles related to the latest cancer research.

Association of Community Cancer Centers
This site provides a database listing of cancer treatment centers in all 50 states. Information describing each center is available here.

CancerGuide
This site was created by a cancer survivor and provides information that helps newly diagnosed cancer patients to make decisions about their treatment. The site provides information on all aspects of cancer care and is very patient oriented.

National Coalition for Cancer Survivorship (NCCS)
1010 Wayne Avenue
5th Floor
Silver Spring, MD 20910
Provides an informational newsletter for cancer survivors.

American Institute for Cancer Research and Nutrition
1-800-843-8114
Provides information on nutrition to prevent cancer.

University of Pennsylvania Cancer Center
Prominent site providing up to date information on the treatment of cancer.

Mayo Clinic Health Oasis
www.mayohealth.org
Mayo Clinic site includes disease and condition reports, health news and features, Ask a Physician, library, and glossary.

InteliHealth
www.intelihealth.com
Johns Hopkins health information center features news and special reports, disease and condition guide, live chat, medical dictionary, physician locator, drug resource center, and newsletter.

American Pain Society

www.ampainsoc.org

More than 3,200 doctors, nurses, scientists, psychologists, and pharmacologists who research and treat pain and act as advocates for patients in pain.

Mayday Pain Resource Center

http://mayday.coh.org

Pain resource center from City of Hope Medical Center, Duarte, CA.

AMA Physician Select

www.ama-assn.org

From the American Medical Association, this site provides information on nearly every licensed physician in the United States.

HospitalSelect

www.hospitalselect.com

A hospital locator, providing information on virtually every hospital in the United States Provided in cooperation with the American Medical Association.

Healthgrades

www.healthgrades.com

Profiles more than 500,000 hospitals and 600,000 physicians.

Clinical Trials

For information on locating clinical trials, you can call the Cancer Information Service of the National Cancer Institute 1-800-4-CANCER (1-800-422-6237); TTY at 1-800-332-8615. The Internet contains many listings of clinical trials at various sites. No specific site lists all of the available trials.

Cancer Care, Inc.

http://www.cancercare.org

This site contains useful general information on clinical trials, including discussions of the pros and cons of participating, reimbursement issues, etc. It is written in an understandable format.

CenterWatch
>http://www.centerwatch.com
>A clinical trials listing service that which provides information on private industry sponsored clinical trials as well as government-sponsored trials.

National Cancer Institute
>The Cancer Information Service provides has information on clinical trials. Call 1-800-4-CANCER (1-800-422-6237); TTY at 1-800-332-8615. Visit CancerNet via the Internet. The URL is http://cancernet.nci.nih.gov. From there, one can access a database called PDQ, a computer system that provides updated information about cancer and cancer treatments.

Glossary

A

Adenocarinoma: The most common type of colorectal cancer.

Adjuvant therapy: Additional therapy given to supplement an initial therapy.

Anemia: Medical term given to the condition of a low red blood count.

Anesthesiologist: Doctor trained in administering anesthesia during surgery.

Anterior-Posterior (AP) Resection: The major curative operation for cancers of the distal rectum.

Antibody: Protein molecule created by the body's immune system to fight foreign substances such as infections.

Anus: Opening at the end of the rectum where stool exits the body.

Ascending Colon: The first part of the colon on the right side of the abdominal cavity.

Astler-Coller: A type of staging system for colorectal cancers.

B

Barium Enema: X-ray test that outlines the colon wall and used to identify polyps.

Benign: Noncancerous.

Bilirubin: Compound made by the liver and involved in digestion of food.

Bladder: Organ, located behind the pubic bone, which collects urine.

Bone Scan: Specialized X-ray test used to evaluate the skeleton for the spread of cancer.

Biopsy: Procedure to surgically remove a piece of tissue for analysis.

Brachytherapy: A form of radiation therapy used to treat cancer.

Coronary Artery: An artery supplying oxygenated blood to the heart.

Cowden's disease: An inherited disease resulting in the formation of colorectal polyps.

CPT-11: A drug given as chemotherapy to treat colorectal cancer.

Coumadin: A drug given to thin the blood.

Crohn's disease: An inflammatory disease of the colon wall resulting in diarrhea and pain.

Cystogram: X-ray test used to evaluate the inside lining of the bladder.

D

Defecation: The act of having a bowel movement.

Demerol: Narcotic drug used to treat pain after surgery.

Descending colon: The part of the colon located on the left side of the abdominal cavity and connecting to the sigmoid colon.

Diarrhea: The passing of liquid stool.

Diverticulosis: A disease of the colon characterized by the formation of small, weak pouches in the wall and resulting in constipation and pain.

Diverticulitis: A disease characterized by infection in the small pouches of diverticulosis.

Duodenum: The name given to the first part of the small intestine leading from the stomach.

Duke's classification: An older staging system, using the letters A, B, C for colorectal cancer.

Dysplastic: Precancerous changes seen in colorectal polyps.

E

E. Coli: A type of bacteria normally found in the colon.

Electrolytes: Blood components of sodium, potassium, chloride, and carbon dioxide.

Endocavity radiation: A type of radiation treatment used to treat cancer.

Endoscopy: The name given to invasive procedures performed to look into a variety of organs in the body.

Enterostomal Nurse: Nurse specializing in the education and care of a colostomy.

Epidural catheter: Small tube inserted at the base of the back for pain control after an operation.

Esophagus: Tube-like organ which carries food from the mouth to the stomach.

External Beam: A type of radiation treatment used to treat cancer.

Extramural: Referring to outside the wall of an organ.

F

Familial Adenomatous Polyposis (FAP): Inherited disease resulting in the formation of thousands of precancerous polyps at an early age.

Fatigue: To be tired.

Fellowship: Name given to the specialized training some doctors acquire after completion of residency.

Fistula: Abnormal connection between two or more hollow organs.

Flatus: Refers to the passing of gas.

Fleets Phosphosoda: Liquid taken by mouth used to clean out the colon before colonoscopy or surgery.

5-Flourouracil (5-FU): Chemotherapy drug used to treat colorectal cancer.

Forceps: Surgical instrument used to grab objects.

G

Gardner's Syndrome: Inherited disease resulting in the formation of precancerous colorectal polyps.

Gastroenterologist: Doctor specializing in treating diseases of the esophagus, stomach, intestine, colon, rectum, and anus.

Gastrointestinal Tract: All-encompassing term given to include the organs involved in eating, digestion, absorption, and waste excretion.

General Anesthesia: Anesthesia given with the purpose of putting patients to sleep during surgery.

General Surgeon: A surgeon qualified to operate on a variety of diseases, including colorectal cancer.

Go-Lytely: Liquid taken by mouth and used to clean out the colon before colonoscopy or surgery.

H

Hematochezia: term used to describe blood-stained stool.

Hematocrit: Red blood cell count given as a percentage.

Hemoglobin: Level of iron present as it relates to red blood cell count.

Hemorrhoids: Abnormal veins located around the anus, causing bleeding and pain.

Hereditary NonPolyposis Colon Cancer (HNPCC): Hereditary disease resulting in the formation of thousands of precancerous polyps at an early age.

Hickman Catheter: Special intravenous device inserted surgically and left in place for the administration of chemotherapy.

Hyperplastic Polyp: A noncancerous polyp.

I

Ileocecal Valve: Valve located at the junction of the small and large intestine.

Ileum: Name given to the last part of the small intestine.

Ileus: The time period when the intestines are inactive after major surgery.

Incentive Spirometer: Plastic device, which patient blow into, after surgery to keep their lungs expanded and prevent pneumonia.

Incision: The surgical site where the actual cutting was performed.

Inflammatory Bowel Disease (IBD): A disease, which is characterized by inflammation of the lining or the entire wall of the colon.

Intravenous: Refers to the inside a vein. Many medications are given this way.

J

Jaundice: A yellowing color of the skin or eyes as a result of a rise in the bilirubin level.

K

L

Laparoscopic Surgery: Surgery performed using small incisions and small instruments.

Lesion: Term given to any abnormal growth anywhere in the body.

Leucovorin: Chemotherapeutic drug taken by mouth to treat colorectal cancer when it has spread to the lymph nodes.

Levamisole: Chemotherapeutic drug taken by mouth to treat colorectal cancer when it has spread to the lymph nodes.

Linear Accelerator: Device that creates the Xray beams used during radiation therapy.

Liver: Largest organ in the abdominal cavity involved in the processing of blood toxins, glucose metabolism, and the digestion of food.

Low Anterior Resection: Major operation performed to treat rectal cancer.

Lymph Node: Pea sized glands located throughout the body and involved in fighting off infection.

M

Magnetic Resonance Imaging (MRI): Specialized X-ray test using electrons to create detailed pictures of the human body.

Malignant Tumor: A tumor that is cancerous and can spread to other parts of the body.

Melena: Medical term for the passing of dark, tarry stools.

Metastasis: The spreading of a cancerous growth to organs in the body.

Minimally Invasive Surgery: Surgery performed using small incisions, fiberoptic cameras, and small surgical instruments.

Morphine: A narcotic drug given intravenously for the control of postoperative pain.

Mucosa: The inner layer of cells lining an organ.

Muscularis Propria: The muscle layer of cells surrounding the mucosa in an organ.

Mutation: A DNA change in a gene resulting in an abnormal functioning and potentially disease.

Myocardial Infarction: The medical term for a heart attack.

N

Nasogastric Tube: A long, clear plastic tube inserted into a patient's stomach during and after surgery to drain any fluid collecting.

Neutropenia: Describes the state of a very low white blood cell count.

O

Oncologist: A doctor specializing in the medical treatment of cancer.

P

Palliative Treatment: Treatment aimed at slowing a disease rather than curing it.

Pathologist: A doctor trained specifically to examine tissue and perform autopsies.

Patient Controlled Anesthesia (PCA): Type of postoperative pain control involving the continuous infusion of intravenous narcotic medicine.

Pericolic Fat: The fat immediately adjacent to the colon wall.

Peritonitis: An acute intra-abdominal infection that has spread to involve the lining of the abdominal cavity.

Peutz-Jegher's Syndrome: An inherited disease resulting in the formation of numerous benign colorectal polyps at an early age.

Pneumatic Compression Stockings: Stockings that periodically contract on the calf muscles during surgery to prevent the formation of blood clots.

Polyp: An abnormal growth that can grow in any organ, especially the colon. Polyps can be benign or malignant.

Portacath: Round device surgically implanted into a large neck vein so chemotherapy can be administered.

Prostate Gland: Walnut-size gland located at the base of the bladder and involved in producing fluid that is part of the male ejaculate.

R

Radiologist: A doctor trained to perform and read all X-rays.

Radiation Oncologist: A doctor trained to perform radiation therapy on patients for the treatment of cancer.

Rectum: The last six inches of colon leading to the anus.

Recurrence: The return of a cancer during the follow-up period after the initial treatment has been carried out.

Red Blood Cells: Cells circulating in the body involved in the metabolism of oxygen and iron.

Resection: To remove surgically.

S

Salmonella: A bacteria that causes food poisoning.

Scleral Icterus: A yellowing of the whites of the eyes due to the buildup of bilirubin in the blood.

Screening: Periodic testing for a specific disease.

Serosa: The outer layer of cells surrounding any organ.

Sessile: Describes the shape of a polyp as being flat and broad-based.

Sigmoid Colon: The part of the colon starting at the end of the left, or descending colon, and connecting to the rectum.

Sigmoidoscopy: Procedure using a lighted scope to examine the sigmoid colon and rectum.

Snare: Wire device used to remove polyps from the colon during a colonoscopy.

Spleen: Organ located beneath the left rib cage and involved in the immune system's ability to fight infection.

Staging: The process of classifying the extent to which a diagnosed cancer has spread.

Submucosa: The layer of cells just beneath the inner lining, or mucosa, of an organ.

Subtotal Colectomy: An operation involving removal of 90 percent of the colon.

Suture: Synthetic material used to sew tissues together.

T

Tenesmus: The sensation of pressure in the rectum immediately after having a bowel movement.

TNM Staging Classification: Universal staging system for cancer used by doctors today describing the extent (T) of the tumor, the nodal (N) involvement, and the presence of metastasis (M).

Total Colectomy: Operation performed to remove the entire colon.

Transrectal Ultrasound: Imaging test using sound waves to evaluate a tumor in the rectum.

Transanal: Refers to any procedure going through the anus.

Transverse Colon: The portion of the colon connecting the right and left colon segments.

Tubular: Referring to the tube-like shape of cells in a some polyps.

Glossary

Turcot's Syndrome: Inherited disease resulting in the formation of numerous colorectal polyps.

Tumor: Tissue growth that can be benign or malignant.

U

Ultrasound: X-ray or imaging test using sound waves to analyze an organ.

V

Versed: A drug used to cause relaxation and sedation before surgery.

Villous: Refers to the microscopic description of a particular polyp.

W

X

Y

Z

Index

Index

Index

vitamins, 112
vomiting, 86

W

warning signs of cancer, 9,
   21–25
weight loss, 22, 25
   after surgery, 73
   as symptom of recurrence, 98
windpipe, 66

X

x-ray, 33, 39, 48, 99
   bones, 37
   chest, 37
   liquid,
   see barium

About the Author

Paul Ruggieri, M.D., a board-certified general surgeon, is chief of the department of surgery at St. Anne's Hospital, Fall River, Massachusetts. He specializes in thyroid and minimally invasive surgery.

Dr. Ruggieri received his medical degree from the Georgetown University School of Medicine in Washington, D.C. He completed his surgical internship and residency at Barnes Hospital, Washington University School of Medicine, St. Louis, Missouri. After his training, he joined the Army and was stationed at the U.S. Army hospital in Fort Polk, Louisiana. During his time in the military, he rose to the rank of major, received the Army Commendation and Meritorious Service Medals, and became the chief of the department of surgery. In 1995, Dr. Ruggieri entered a private surgical practice near Nashville, Tennessee. In 1998, he returned to his native New England to join a surgical group in southeastern Massachusetts.

Dr. Ruggieri is a fellow in the American College of Surgeons and is a member of the Society of American Gastrointestinal Endoscopic Surgeons. He is also the author of *The Surgery Handbook—A Guide to Understanding Your Operation* (Addicus Books, 1999).

Addicus Books Consumer Health Titles

Cancers of the Mouth and Throat — A Patient's Guide to Treatment   *$14.95*
    William Lydiatt, MD; Perry Johnson, MD / 1-886039-44-5

Colon & Rectal Cancer—A Patient's Guide to Treatment   *$14.95*
    Paul Ruggieri, MD / 1-886039-51-8

Coping with Psoriasis—A Patient's Guide to Treatment   *$14.95*
    David L. Cram, MD / 1-886039-47-X

The Healing Touch—
Keeping the Doctor/Patient Relationship Alive Under Managed Care   *$9.95*
    David Cram, MD / 1-886039-31-3

Living with P.C.O.S.—Polycystic Ovarian Syndrome   *$14.95*
    Angela Boss; Evelina Sterling / 1-886039-49-6

Lung Cancer—A Guide to Treatment & Diagnosis   *$14.95*
    Walter J. Scott, MD / 1-886039-43-7

The Macular Degeneration Source Book   *$14.95*
    Bert Glaser, MD, Lester Picker / 1-886039-53-4 (Fall 2001)

Overcoming Postpartum Depression and Anxiety   *$12.95*
    Linda Sebastian, RN / 1-886930-34-8

Prescription Drug Abuse—The Hidden Epidemic   *$14.95*
    Rod Colvin / 1-886039-22-4

Simple Changes: The Boomer's Guide to a Healthier, Happier Life   *$9.95*
    L. Joe Porter, MD / 1-886039-35-6

Straight Talk About Breast Cancer   *$12.95*
    Suzanne Braddock, MD / 1-886039-21-6

The Stroke Recovery Book   *$14.95*
    Kip Burkman, MD / 1-886039-30-5

The Surgery Handbook—A Guide to Understanding Your Operation   *$14.95*
    Paul Ruggieri, MD / 1-886039-38-0

Understanding Parkinson's Disease—A Self-Help Guide   *$14.95*
    David Cram, MD / 1-886039-40-2

Please send:

_____ copies of _____
(Title of book)

at $ _____ each   TOTAL: _____

Nebr. residents add 5% sales tax   _____

Shipping/Handling
    $4.00 for first book.
    $1.10 for each additional book   _____

TOTAL ENCLOSED: _____

Name _____

Address _____

City _____ State _____ Zip _____

❑ **Visa**   ❑ **MasterCard**   ❑ **American Express**

Credit card number _____ Expiration date _____

Order by credit card, personal check or money order. Send to:

Addicus Books
Mail Order Dept.
P.O. Box 45327
Omaha, NE 68145
Or, order **TOLL FREE: 800-352-2873**
or online at
www.AddicusBooks.com

OCT 2 5 2001

14 DAY

DATE DUE

GAYLORD			PRINTED IN U.S.A